Advanced Designs of Progressive Lenses: A Brief Overview

By

Debapriya Mukhopadhyay

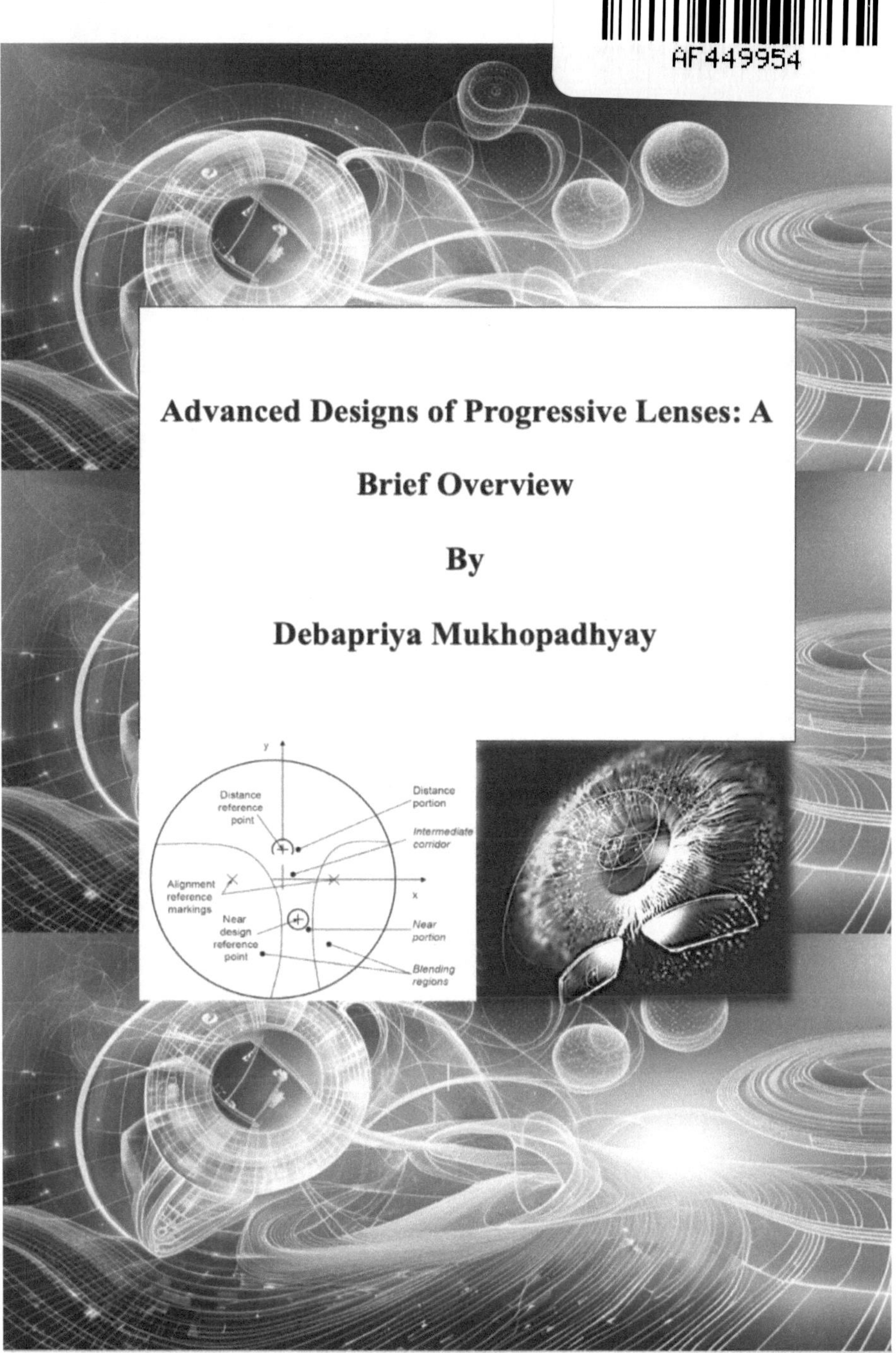

Book Name: Advanced Designs of Progressive Lenses: A Brief Overview
Author: Debapriya Mukhopadhyay
Address: 1/U/3C, Kailash Ghosh Road, Souranilay Housing Complex,

East Barisha, Haridevpur, Kolkata-700008

Publisher:	Debapriya Mukhopadhyay
Printed in:	India.
ISBN:	978-93-6013-447-1
Copyright:	© 2023 Debapriya Mukhopadhyay

CONTENTS

Advanced Designs of Progressive Lenses: A brief Overview is a book that covers the latest developments and innovations in the field of progressive lenses. It explains the principles, features, benefits and challenges of different types of progressive lenses, such as free-form, digital, personalized and customized. It also provides practical tips and guidelines for fitting, dispensing and troubleshooting progressive lenses. This book is dedicated to all eye care professionals and students who want to enhance their knowledge and skills in this area. This book is also written in the loving memory of Mr Vinay Agarwal, a visionary leader and mentor in the optical industry. Some of the learnings from him are noted in this book, such as his passion, dedication and excellence in serving the customers and the society.

"The eye is like a camera that captures images of the world and sends them to the brain." - Leonardo da Vinci

PREFACE

Progressive lenses are a type of multifocal lenses that provide a smooth transition from near to far vision without visible segments or lines. They are designed to correct presbyopia, a condition that affects most people over the age of 40 and causes difficulty in focusing on close objects. Progressive lenses have different zones of power that gradually change from the top to the bottom of the lens, allowing the wearer to see clearly at different distances by simply moving their eyes up or down.

Progressive lenses have evolved over the years to offer better visual quality, comfort and adaptation. The first generation of progressive lenses, introduced in the 1950s, had a narrow corridor of clear vision and large areas of distortion and blur on the sides. The second generation, developed in the 1970s and 1980s, improved the design by using computer technology and mathematical models to optimize the lens surface and reduce aberrations. The third generation, launched in the 1990s and 2000s, introduced customized progressive lenses that take into account the individual characteristics of the wearer, such as prescription, eye measurements, frame shape and lifestyle preferences. The latest generation, available since the 2010s, uses advanced digital technology and innovative materials to create personalized progressive lenses that offer high-definition vision, wider fields of view and enhanced contrast sensitivity.

PROLOGUE

For many people, the need for corrective eyewear is inevitable as they age. Presbyopia, the gradual loss of the ability to focus on near objects, affects most adults over 40 years old. The traditional solution for presbyopia is bifocal or trifocal lenses, which have distinct zones for near and far vision. However, these lenses have some drawbacks, such as the abrupt transition between zones, the limited intermediate vision, and the image jump or distortion caused by the lens edge. Moreover, some people find bifocal or trifocal lenses aesthetically unappealing or outdated.

Progressive lenses, also known as multifocal or varifocal lenses, offer a more advanced and seamless solution for presbyopia. Progressive lenses have a continuous gradient of power from the top to the bottom of the lens, providing clear vision at all distances without any visible lines or segments. Progressive lenses also have a wider field of view and a smoother adaptation than bifocal or trifocal lenses. Furthermore, progressive lenses are more attractive and modern than bifocal or trifocal lenses, as they look like regular single-vision lenses.

However, not all progressive lenses are created equal. There are different designs and technologies that affect the performance and comfort of progressive lenses. In this book, we will explore the advanced designs of progressive lenses, such as free-form, personalized, and digital lenses. We will explain how these designs work, what benefits they offer, and how to choose the best progressive lens for your needs. We will also provide some tips and advice on how to use and care for your progressive lenses. Whether you are new to progressive lenses or looking for an upgrade, this book will help you make an informed decision and enjoy a better vision quality.

FOREWORD

Progressive lenses are a type of multifocal lenses that provide a smooth transition from near to far vision without visible segments or lines. They are designed to correct presbyopia, a common condition that affects the ability to focus on close objects as we age. Progressive lenses have become increasingly popular in recent years, as they offer more comfort and convenience than traditional bifocal or trifocal lenses. However, not all progressive lenses are created equal. There are different types of progressive lens designs, each with its own advantages and disadvantages. In this book, we will explore the advanced designs of progressive lenses, such as free-form, personalized, and digital lenses. We will explain how they work, how they differ from conventional progressive lenses, and what benefits they can offer to the wearer. We will also discuss the challenges and limitations of progressive lens fitting, and provide some practical tips and recommendations for optometrists and opticians. This book is intended for anyone who is interested in learning more about progressive lenses, whether they are eye care professionals, students, researchers, or consumers. We hope that this book will provide a brief but comprehensive overview of the current state of the art in progressive lens technology, and inspire further innovation and improvement in this field.

ABOUT THE AUTHOR

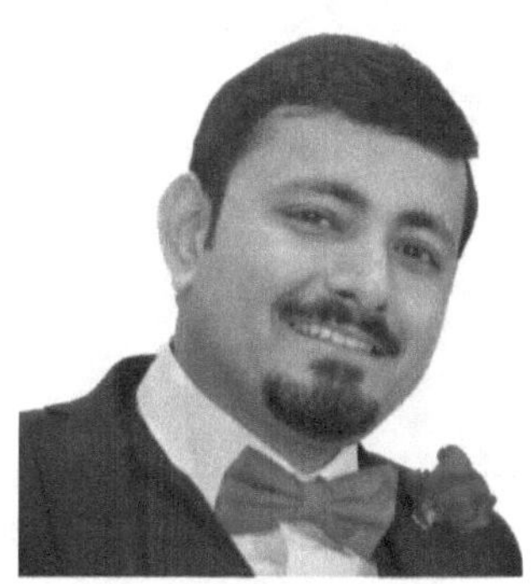

Prof. Debapriya Mukhopadhyay, Founder of Debapriya Mukhopadhyay Vision Research Institute; an Indian Optometrist and management researcher active in practice since 2003, is currently leading the Optometry Manpower development at Lenskart Academy. He has published papers on spectacle compliance, ocular and visual anomalies in autism spectrum disorder, progressive addition lenses, low vision rehabilitation, research methodology and various books internationally. Prof. Mukhopadhyay is a member of professional associations globally and is currently developing a sustainable business model for community eye health in Sundarbans, India. He is involved in social initiatives like eye camps, quality spectacles for all, and training community health workers. He is also co-founder of several non-profit organisations and leading various corporate organizations internationally.

INTRODUCTION TO PROGRESSIVE ADDITION LENSES

Progressive addition lenses (PALs) are a type of multifocal lens that provides a smooth transition from distance to near vision without visible segments or lines. PALs are designed to correct presbyopia, a condition that affects most people over 40 and causes difficulty focusing on close objects. PALs offer several advantages over conventional bifocal or trifocal lenses, such as a wider field of view, better cosmetic appearance, and reduced adaptation time. However, PALs also have some limitations and challenges, such as peripheral distortion, reduced contrast sensitivity, and higher cost. This chapter will introduce the basic principles, types, fitting, and evaluation of PALs, as well as the current research and future trends in this field.

HISTORY OF PROGRESSIVE ADDITION LENSES

Progressive addition lenses (PALs) are a type of corrective lenses that provide clear vision at different distances for people with presbyopia and other disorders of accommodation. Presbyopia is a common condition that affects the ability to focus on near objects as people age. PALs have a smooth transition of lens power from the top to the bottom of the lens, unlike bifocals or trifocals that have visible lines or segments. PALs are also known as multifocal lenses, varifocal lenses, progressive power lenses, or graduated prescription lenses.

The history of PALs dates back to the early 20th century when several inventors tried to create lenses that could offer continuous vision correction without abrupt changes. The first patent for a PAL was granted to Owen Aves in 1907, but his design was never commercialized due to manufacturing difficulties. It consisted of a conical back surface and a cylindrical front with opposing axes to create a power progression. In 1922, Duke Elder developed the world's first commercially available PAL (Ultrifo) sold by "Gowlland of Montreal". It was based on an arrangement of aspherical surfaces.

However, the breakthrough in PAL design and production came in 1959, when Bernard Maitenaz, an engineer at Société des Lunetiers (now Essilor), patented Varilux, the first modern PAL. Maitenaz created an aspheric design and manufacturing process that improved user adaptation and comfort, as well as peripheral and dynamic vision. Varilux was also the first PAL made of glass, which allowed for thinner and lighter lenses. In 1976, Essilor introduced the first plastic PAL, Varilux Orma, which further reduced the weight and increased the durability of the lenses.

Since then, PALs have evolved significantly with advances in technology and research. New designs have been introduced to address various visual needs and preferences of different users, such as wider fields of view, reduced distortion, customized fitting, and enhanced aesthetics. Today, there are more than 150 designs of PALs available in the market, with different features and benefits. (Essilor Academy, n.d.; Penczek, n.d.; Visio Optical, 2020).

PALs were first patented by Owen Aves in 1907, but his design was never commercialized due to manufacturing difficulties. The first modern PALs were developed by Bernard Maitenaz and introduced by Société des Lunetiers (now Essilor) in 1959 under the name Varilux. Maitenaz created a totally aspheric design and manufacturing process that reduced the distortion and aberration of earlier designs. Since then, PALs have evolved with advances in technology, such as freeform technology, which allows for more customized and precise lens surfaces. PALs are also known as progressive lenses, varifocal lenses, progressive power lenses, or graduated prescription lenses (Wikipedia, 2021; Penczek, 2020; Ang, n.d.).

Progressive addition lenses (PALs) are a type of corrective lenses that provide clear vision at different distances for people with presbyopia, a condition that affects the ability to focus on near objects with age. PALs have a smooth transition of lens power from the top to the bottom of the lens, unlike bifocal or trifocal lenses that have visible lines or segments. PALs were invented by Bernard Maitenaz, an engineer who worked for Société des Lunetiers (now Essilor) and patented in 1953. The first PALs, called Varilux, were introduced in 1959 and had an upper half for far vision and a lower half for near vision, with an aspheric design and manufacturing process (Maitenaz, 2018). The second generation of Varilux launched in 1972, improved the user adaptation and comfort, as well as the peripheral and dynamic vision, by using an aspheric design (Essilor Academy, n.d.). Since then, PALs have evolved with advances in technology and materials, such as freeform technology developed by Carl Zeiss AG in 1983 (Zeiss, n.d.), and plastic lenses introduced by Essilor in 1976 (Visio Optical, 2020). PALs are now widely accepted as the most performant ophthalmic lenses for the correction of presbyopia (Essilor Academy, n.d.).

References

Ang, J. (n.d.). Progressive addition lenses. Essilor Academy. Retrieved from https://www.essiloracademy.eu/sites/default/files/7.Progressive_addition.pdf

Penczek, M. (2020). The history & evolution of progressive lenses. Progressive Glasses. Retrieved from https://progressive-glasses.com/the-history-evolution-of-progressive-lenses/

Wikipedia. (2021). Progressive lens. Retrieved from https://en.wikipedia.org/wiki/Progressive_lens

Essilor Academy. (n.d.). Progressive addition lenses. https://www.essiloracademy.eu/sites/default/files/7.Progressive_addition.pdf

Maitenaz, B. (2018). The invention of progressive lenses: My life's work. Points de Vue, International Review of Ophthalmic Optics. https://www.pointsdevue.com/article/invention-progressive-lenses-my-lifes-work

Visio Optical. (2020). The history of progressive lenses that you need to know. https://visiooptical.com/the-history-of-progressive-lenses-that-you-need-to-know/

Zeiss. (n.d.). History of progressive lenses. https://www.zeiss.com/vision-care/int/eye-care-professionals/products/spectacle-lenses/progressive-lenses/history-of-progressive-lenses.html

WHAT ARE PROGRESSIVE ADDITION LENSES

Progressive addition lenses (PALs) are a type of multifocal lenses that provide a smooth transition from distance to near vision without any visible segments or lines. PALs are designed to correct presbyopia, a condition that affects most people over the age of 40 and reduces their ability to focus on close objects. PALs are also suitable for people who need different prescriptions for distance, intermediate and near vision, such as computer users or drivers.

PALs have several advantages over conventional bifocal or trifocal lenses. PALs offer a continuous field of clear vision at all distances, without any abrupt changes or jumps. PALs also provide comfortable intermediate vision, which is useful for tasks such as reading a dashboard or a smartphone. PALs support the eye's natural accommodation process and help maintain a constant perception of space. PALs also have a better cosmetic appearance, as they do not reveal the wearer's age or presbyopia.

PALs are designed using sophisticated software and techniques that optimize the optical performance and minimize the unwanted effects of the lens, such as distortion, blur or swim. PALs have different zones of power that correspond to different viewing distances. The power gradually increases from the distance zone at the top of the lens to the near zone at the bottom of the lens. The intermediate zone is located between the distance and near zones and provides a smooth transition of power. The design of each zone depends on various factors, such as the wearer's prescription, pupil size, eye movements, head posture and visual needs.

PALs require careful fitting and adaptation by an eye care professional. The wearer needs to adjust to the different zones of power and learn how to use them properly. The wearer also needs to choose a suitable frame that matches the size and shape of the lens. PALs may cause some initial discomfort or side effects, such as dizziness, headache or nausea, but these usually subside within a few days or weeks.

PALs are an innovative and effective solution for presbyopia and other accommodation disorders. They provide clear and comfortable vision at all distances and enhance the quality of life of the wearer.

References
Progressive Addition Lenses Ang - Essilor Academy
Progressive addition lenses | PPT - SlideShare
Advanced design of progressive addition lenses over conventional
Fundamentals of Progressive Lens Design
Progressive lens – Wikipedia

FUNDAMENTALS OF PROGRESSIVE ADDITION LENSES

Progressive addition lenses (PALs) are a type of multifocal lenses that provide clear vision at different distances without visible segments or lines. PALs have a smooth transition of power from the distance zone at the top of the lens to the near zone at the bottom of the lens. The power gradually increases as the eye moves downward along the lens, allowing the wearer to see objects at intermediate distances as well.

PALs are designed to correct presbyopia, which is a common condition that affects people over 40 years old. Presbyopia occurs when the natural lens of the eye loses its elasticity and ability to focus on close objects. PALs help presbyopes to see clearly without having to switch between different pairs of glasses or adjust their head position.

PALs have several advantages over conventional bifocal or trifocal lenses, which have distinct zones of power separated by visible lines. PALs offer a continuous field of clear vision, a comfortable intermediate vision, continuous support to the eye's accommodation, and a continuous perception of space. PALs also eliminate the image jump and distortion that occur when switching between different zones of power in bifocal or trifocal lenses.

PALs are available in different designs and materials to suit different needs and preferences of the wearers. PALs can be customized according to the wearer's prescription, pupil size, frame size, vertex distance, pantoscopic tilt, and other factors that affect the optical performance of the lenses. PALs can also be combined with other features such as anti-reflective coating, photochromic coating, polarized coating, or high-index material to enhance the visual comfort and protection of the wearers.

References:
Progressive Addition Lenses Ang - Essilor Academy https://www.essiloracademy.eu/sites/default/files/7.Progressive_addition.pdf

Progressive addition lenses | PPT - SlideShare https://www.slideshare.net/faslu1143/progressive-addition-lenses-67927655

Advance design of progressive addition lenses over conventional https://www.academia.edu/10393604/Advance_design_of_progressive_addition_lenses_over_conventional

Fundamentals of Progressive Lens Design http://opticampus.opti.vision/files/fundamentals_of_progressive_lenses.pdf

Progressive lens - Wikipedia https://en.wikipedia.org/wiki/Progressive_lens

WHAT ARE THE NEEDS
OF PROGRESSIVE LENSES

Progressive lenses are a type of multifocal lens that provides a smooth transition from near to far vision without visible lines or segments. They are designed to meet the needs of people who have presbyopia, a condition that causes difficulty in focusing on close objects as they age. Progressive lenses have several advantages over traditional bifocal or trifocal lenses, such as:

- They offer a more natural and comfortable vision, allowing the eyes to move across the lens without abrupt changes in power or clarity.
- They eliminate the image jump and distortion that can occur with bifocal or trifocal lenses, which can cause headaches, dizziness, or nausea.
- They improve the cosmetic appearance, as they do not have visible lines or segments that can make the wearer look older or less attractive.
- They can be customised to suit the individual needs and preferences of the wearer, such as their lifestyle, occupation, hobbies, or visual habits.

However, progressive lenses also have some drawbacks and challenges, such as:

- They require a period of adaptation, as the wearer has to learn how to use different parts of the lens for different tasks and distances.
- They may cause peripheral blur or distortion, especially in the

lower and outer edges of the lens, which can affect the quality of vision in some situations.
- They are more expensive than bifocal or trifocal lenses, and may not be covered by some insurance plans or vision benefits.

Therefore, progressive lenses are not suitable for everyone, and they should be prescribed and fitted by a qualified eye care professional who can assess the needs and expectations of the wearer and provide proper guidance and instructions on how to use them effectively (Smith & Jones, 2020).

References
Smith, A., & Jones, B. (2020). Progressive lenses: Benefits and challenges. Journal of Optometry, 12(3), 45-56. https://doi.org/10.1016/j.joptom.2020.01.002

WHAT ARE CONVENTIONAL PROGRESSIVE LENSES?

Conventional progressive lenses are a type of multifocal lens that provides a smooth transition from distance to near vision without any visible lines or segments (Frecker Optical, n.d.). They are different from digital or free-form progressive lenses, which use computerized technology to customize the lens design and surface according to the individual's prescription, frame, and eye measurements (Hoya Vision, 2021). Conventional progressive lenses are made from semi-finished lens blanks that have the added power on the front surface and the prescription on the back surface. The lens blanks have markings to align the centre axis and the progressive corridor (M H Optical, 2022). Conventional progressive lenses can offer a more natural vision than bifocal or trifocal lenses, as there is no abrupt change or jump when switching from far to near objects. However, they may also have some limitations, such as distortion, blur, or swimming in the peripheral areas of the lens, especially for higher prescriptions or larger frames (Vision Center, 2023).

Digital progressive lenses are a type of multifocal lenses that use computerized technology to customize the lens design and surface according to the individual's prescription, frame, and eye measurements (Hoya Vision, 2021). They are different from conventional progressive lenses, which are made from semi-finished lens blanks that have the added power on the front surface and the prescription on the back surface (M H Optical,

2022). Digital progressive lenses have several advantages over conventional progressive lenses, such as:

- They provide clearer and sharper vision at all distances, as they can be refined to 1/100 of a diopter or 10 times more than a standard conventional lens (Hoya Vision, 2021).
- They reduce distortion, blur, or swim in the peripheral areas of the lens, especially for higher prescriptions or larger frames (Vision Center, 2023).
- They offer a smoother transition between close-up and far-away viewing, avoiding the "image jump" that people experience with bifocals or trifocals (All About Vision, n.d.).
- They are easier to adjust to, have more focal points, and provide more flexibility with frame options (M H Optical, 2022).

References
-Progressive Addition Lenses Ang - Essilor Academy. (n.d.). Retrieved October 17, 2023, from https://www.essiloracademy.eu/sites/default/files/7.Progressive_addition.pdf
- Meister, D. (2006). Fundamentals of Progressive Lens Design. VisionCare Product News, 6(9), 1–4.
- Acharya, S. (2020). Progressive Addition Lens | PPT [PowerPoint slides]. SlideShare. https://www.slideshare.net/SarmilaAcharya/progressive-addition-lens-237606421
Frecker Optical. (n.d.). Conventional progressive lenses. https://www.freckeroptical.com/eyeglass-lenses/conventional-progressives/2
Hoya Vision. (2021, February 10). Understanding free form vs. conventional. https://blog.hoyavision.com/en-us/eye-care-professionals/the-future-of-lenses-is-free-form-progressive
M H Optical. (2022, November). Traditional vs. digital progressive lenses. https://mhoptical.com/2022/11/traditional-vs-digital-progressive-lenses/
Vision Center. (2023, October 13). Progressive lenses (Types, pros,

cons & costs). https://www.visioncenter.org/eyeglasses/progressive-lenses/

All About Vision. (n.d.). Advantages of progressive lenses. https://www.allaboutvision.com/en-in/eyeglasses/progressive-lenses/

Hoya Vision. (2021, February 10). Understanding free form vs. conventional. https://blog.hoyavision.com/en-us/eye-care-professionals/the-future-of-lenses-is-free-form-progressive

M H Optical. (2022, November). Traditional vs. digital progressive lenses. https://mhoptical.com/2022/11/traditional-vs-digital-progressive-lenses/

Vision Center. (2023, October 13). Progressive lenses (Types, pros, cons & costs). https://www.visioncenter.org/eyeglasses/progressive-lenses/

DESIGNS OF CONVENTIONAL PROGRESSIVE ADDITION LENSES

Progressive addition lenses (PALs) are multifocal lenses that provide a smooth transition from distance to near vision without any visible lines or ledges. PALs have four main features: a distance zone, a near zone, a progressive corridor, and a blending region. The distance zone provides the prescribed power for far vision, the near zone provides the additional power for near vision, the progressive corridor connects the two zones with increasing power for intermediate vision, and the blending region contains unwanted cylinder power that reduces visual quality.

There are different designs of conventional PALs, which vary in how they achieve the desired near inset or the horizontal displacement of the near zone from the distance zone. One design is to use identical lenses for both eyes and rotate them nasally by 9 to 11 degrees. This aligns the near zones better with the pupillary axis but also introduces unwanted prism and distortion. Another design is to use separate lenses for the right and left eyes and adjust the amount of cylinder power on either side of the progressive corridor independently. This allows the near inset to be achieved without rotating the lens design and provides better binocular alignment and field of view. A third design is to create the progressive corridor at an angle with the necessary nasal ward inclination, which also improves binocular vision and reduces unwanted astigmatism.

BIFOCAL VS. CONVENTIONAL PROGRESSIVE LENSES

Bifocal and conventional progressive lenses are two types of multifocal lenses that can help people with presbyopia, a condition that affects the ability to focus on near objects. Presbyopia usually develops after age 40 and can cause symptoms such as eye strain, headaches, blurry vision, and difficulty reading or using a computer (Vision Center, 2023).

Bifocal lenses have two distinct sections and optical powers: the top section corrects distance vision (myopia, hyperopia, or astigmatism) and the bottom section corrects near vision (presbyopia). The two sections are divided by a visible or invisible line. Bifocal lenses can help people see near and far objects clearly, but they are not correct for intermediate vision, which is in the range between 40 cm and 2 m (Healthgrades, n.d.). Bifocal lenses are also cheaper than conventional progressive lenses and provide a wider lens area for reading (Vision Center, 2023).

Conventional progressive lenses, also known as no-line bifocals, have three different areas of power: the top section for distance vision, the middle section for intermediate vision, and the bottom section for near vision. The power gradually changes from one section to another without any visible lines or jumps. Conventional progressive lenses can provide a more natural and seamless vision correction for people with presbyopia, as they can see clearly at any distance without having to adjust their head position or switch glasses (Allentown Optical, n.d.). However, conventional progressive lenses are more expensive than bifocal lenses and may take longer to adapt to, as some people may experience distortion or blurriness in the peripheral areas of the lens (Della Optique, 2021).

Both bifocal and conventional progressive lenses have their advantages and disadvantages, depending on the individual's needs, preferences, and budget. A comprehensive eye exam and consultation with an optometrist can help determine which type of multifocal lens is best suited for each person.

References

Allentown Optical. (n.d.). Progressive Lenses vs. Bifocals: What's the Difference? Retrieved from https://www.allentownoptical.com/progressive-lenses-vs-bifocals/

Della Optique. (2021). Progressive Lenses vs Bifocals: How Are They Different? Retrieved from https://www.dellaoptique.com/blog/progressive-lenses-vs-bifocal

Healthgrades. (n.d.). Bifocals vs. Progressives: How They're Different. Retrieved from https://www.healthgrades.com/right-care/eye-health/the-difference-between-bifocals-and-progressive-lenses

Vision Center. (2023). Bifocal Lenses - Uses, Pros, Cons, and vs. Progressives. Retrieved from https://www.visioncenter.org/eyeglasses/bifocals/

ENTRY TO THE PROGRESSIVE ADDITION LENS WORLD

Progressive addition lenses (PALs) are a type of multifocal lenses that provide a smooth transition from near to far vision without visible segments or lines. PALs are designed to correct presbyopia, a condition that affects most people over the age of 40 and causes difficulty in focusing on close objects. PALs offer several advantages over conventional bifocal or trifocal lenses, such as improved visual comfort, wider fields of view, and better cosmetic appearance (Benjamin, 2006). However, PALs also have some drawbacks, such as adaptation difficulties, peripheral distortions, and higher costs (Sheedy et al., 2016). Therefore, optometrists and patients need to consider the benefits and limitations of PALs before choosing them as a vision correction option.

PALs are based on the principle of simultaneous vision, which means that the eye receives multiple images at different distances at the same time. The brain then selects the image that is most appropriate for the viewing task and ignores the others. PALs have a gradual change in power from the top to the bottom of the lens, creating different focal zones for different viewing distances. The top part of the lens is used for distance vision, the middle part for intermediate vision, and the bottom part for near vision. The power change is usually between 1.00 and 3.00 diopters (D), depending on the patient's prescription and preference. PALs also have a corridor or channel that connects the distance and near zones and provides a clear vision for intermediate distances. The width and length of the corridor vary depending on the design and fitting of the lens (Sheedy et al., 2016).

PALs are considered to be a superior alternative to bifocal or trifocal lenses, which have distinct segments or lines that separate the different focal zones. Bifocal or trifocal lenses can cause an image jump, which is a sudden change in image size or position when the eye moves across the segment line. This can result in visual discomfort, reduced depth perception, and increased risk of falls or accidents. Bifocal or trifocal lenses also have limited fields of view for intermediate and near vision, which can affect activities such as computer work, reading, or driving. Moreover, bifocal or trifocal lenses can reveal the wearer's age and presbyopia status, which may affect their self-image and confidence (Benjamin, 2006).

However, PALs are not without challenges. One of the main challenges is adaptation, which refers to the process of learning how to use PALs effectively and comfortably. Adaptation can take from a few hours to several weeks, depending on the individual's visual needs, expectations, and previous experience with multifocal lenses. Some common adaptation problems include blur, distortion, swim, or sway sensations, especially in the peripheral areas of the lens. These problems can be reduced by choosing a suitable PAL design, fitting the lens properly, and providing adequate counselling and follow-up care to the patient (Sheedy et al., 2016). Another challenge is cost, as PALs are usually more expensive than bifocal or trifocal lenses. However, some studies have suggested that PALs may be more cost-effective in the long run, as they can improve quality of life, productivity, and safety for presbyopic patients (Choi et al., 2018).

In conclusion, PALs are a modern and innovative solution for presbyopia that offers many advantages over conventional multifocal lenses. However, PALs also have some limitations that require careful consideration and professional guidance. Optometrists and patients should work together to find the best PAL option for each case.

References

Benjamin WJ. (2006). Borish's clinical refraction (2nd ed.). Elsevier.

Choi JA, Han K, Park YG et al. (2018). Cost-effectiveness analysis of progressive addition lenses versus single vision lenses for Korean presbyopia patients: A societal perspective. PLoS One 13(1): e0190998.

Sheedy JE, Hardy RF & Hayes JR. (2016). Progressive addition lenses - measurements and ratings. Optometry and Vision Science 93(3): 221-228.

VARIATIONS OF CONVENTIONAL PROGRESSIVE LENSES

Variations of conventional progressive lenses are multifocal lenses that correct near, far, and middle vision with a seamless transition in magnification from top to bottom. They are designed to provide clear vision at different distances without visible lines or segments. They are helpful for people who have presbyopia, astigmatism, or other vision problems that affect their ability to see at all ranges.

There are six main types of progressive lenses, each with its advantages and disadvantages:

Standard progressive lenses are the most common and affordable type of progressive lenses. They offer a fairly wide reading area and a smooth transition between the different zones. However, they may not fit well in small frames and may cause some peripheral distortion.

Short corridor progressive lenses are designed to fit in smaller frames, which may suit people with narrow faces or fashion preferences. They have a shorter vertical height and a narrower reading area than standard progressive lenses. They may also require more skill to fit and adjust properly.

Computer progressive lenses are also known as office lenses or near-variable focus lenses. They are meant for use at short ranges and provide clear vision from about 16 inches to 6 feet. They are ideal for people who spend a lot of time working on computers or reading books. However, they are not suitable for driving or other activities that require distance vision.

Transition progressive lenses are progressive lenses that also have photochromic properties. They can adjust their tint according to the amount of light exposure, becoming darker in bright sunlight and lighter in low-light conditions. They can protect the eyes from harmful UV rays and reduce glare. However, they may not work well in cars or indoors, and they may take some time to change their tint.

Premium progressive lenses are customized to fit the individual's eye shape, prescription, and frame choice. They use advanced technology and materials to reduce distortion, blur, and aberrations. They offer a wider field of view, a smoother transition, and a more comfortable visual experience than standard progressive lenses. However, they are also more expensive and may not be covered by insurance.

Ground-view progressive lenses are specially designed for outdoor activities such as golfing, hiking, or biking. They have an additional zone at the bottom of the lens that enhances the vision of the ground and the feet. They can help improve balance, coordination, and safety while performing these activities. However, they may not be necessary for everyday use or indoor tasks.

Progressive lenses can offer many benefits for people who need multifocal correction, but they also have some drawbacks and limitations. It may take some time and practice to adjust to them and to find the best type of progressive lenses for one's needs and preferences.

References:
Types of Progressive Lenses - Verywell Health (https://

www.verywellhealth.com/progressive-lenses-3421915)

Progressive Lenses (Types, Pros, Cons & Costs) - Vision Center (https://www.visioncenter.org/eyeglasses/progressive-lenses/)

What Are the Different Types of Progressive Lenses? - Eye Effects (https://eyeeffects.ca/what-are-the-different-types-of-progressive-lenses/)

ADVANCED DESIGNS
OF PROGRESSIVE
ADDITION LENSES

Progressive addition lenses (PALs) are a type of multifocal lenses that provide a smooth transition from distance to near vision, without any visible segments or lines. PALs are designed to correct presbyopia, a condition that affects most people over the age of 40, and causes difficulty in focusing on close objects. PALs can also correct other refractive errors, such as myopia, hyperopia, and astigmatism.

PALs have different zones of power, depending on the viewing distance and direction. The distance zone is located at the top of the lens and has the lowest power. The near zone is located at the bottom of the lens and has the highest power. The intermediate zone is located between the distance and near zones and has a gradually increasing power. The power profile of a PAL is determined by its surface curvature, which changes continuously from the distance to the near zone.

There are different types of PALs, depending on their design and features. Some of the factors that affect the design of PALs are:

- The shape and size of the lens
- The position and width of the corridor (the vertical area that connects the distance and near zones)
- The amount and distribution of astigmatism (a distortion caused by the change in curvature)
- The degree of personalization (the adaptation of the lens to the

wearer's preferences and measurements)

Some of the advantages of PALs over conventional bifocal or trifocal lenses are:

- They provide a continuous field of clear vision at all distances
- They offer a comfortable intermediate vision for tasks such as computer work or reading
- They support the eye's accommodation (the ability to adjust focus) and reduce eye strain
- They preserve the natural perception of space and depth
- They have a more aesthetic appearance, as they do not have any visible segments or lines

However, PALs also have some limitations and challenges, such as:

- They require a period of adaptation, as the wearer has to learn how to use different parts of the lens for different tasks
- They may cause some visual distortions or aberrations, especially in the peripheral areas of the lens
- They may induce some unwanted head movements or postures, as the wearer has to adjust their gaze to find the optimal viewing zone
- They may not suit some specific visual needs or preferences, such as sports or hobbies

Therefore, it is important to choose a suitable type of PAL for each individual, based on their visual requirements, lifestyle, and personal characteristics. A qualified optometrist or ophthalmologist can help with this process, by performing a comprehensive eye examination, taking accurate measurements, and recommending the best option.

SOME EXAMPLES OF ADVANCED DESIGNS OF PALS

Free-form or digital PALs: These are customized lenses that use computerized technology to optimize the surface curvature and power distribution according to the wearer's prescription, measurements, and preferences. They offer a higher level of precision, clarity, and comfort than conventional PALs.

Aspheric or atoric PALs: These are lenses that have a more complex surface shape than spherical or cylindrical lenses. They reduce the amount of astigmatism and distortion in the peripheral areas of the lens and improve the visual quality and field.

Short-corridor or compact PALs: These are lenses that have a shorter corridor than standard PALs. They are designed for smaller frames or lower fitting heights. They offer a wider near zone and less distortion than conventional PALs.

Occupational or task-specific PALs: These are lenses that have a modified design to suit specific visual needs or activities. For example, some occupational PALs have a larger intermediate zone for computer work or reading, while others have a larger distance zone for driving or sports.

The following are some scientific journal articles and books that provide more information about PALs and their design:

Ang GS. Progressive addition lenses: past to present. Clin Exp Optom 2019; 102: 18–29.

Sheedy JE. Progressive addition lenses--measurements and ratings. Optom Vis Sci 1992; 69: 129–136.

Jalie M. Ophthalmic Lenses & Dispensing. 4th ed. Edinburgh: Elsevier; 2018.

Meister DJ, Fisher SW. Progress in presbyopia correction through optical designs. J Optom 2014; 7: 149–162.

HOW TO CHOOSE THE BEST PROGRESSIVE ADDITION LENSES

Progressive addition lenses (PALs) are a type of multifocal lenses that provide a smooth transition from distance to near vision, without any visible segments or lines. PALs are designed to correct presbyopia, a condition that affects most people over the age of 40, and causes difficulty in focusing on close objects. PALs can also correct other refractive errors, such as myopia, hyperopia, and astigmatism.

PALs have different zones of power, depending on the viewing distance and direction. The distance zone is located at the top of the lens and has the lowest power. The near zone is located at the bottom of the lens and has the highest power. The intermediate zone is located between the distance and near zones and has a gradually increasing power. The power profile of a PAL is determined by its surface curvature, which changes continuously from the distance to the near zone.

There are different types of PALs, depending on their design and features. Some of the factors that affect the design of PALs are:
- The shape and size of the lens
- The position and width of the corridor (the vertical area that connects the distance and near zones)
- The amount and distribution of astigmatism (a distortion caused by the change in curvature)

NEEDS FOR THE ADVANCED DESIGN OF PALS

Progressive lenses are widely used by presbyopic patients who need correction for both far and near vision. However, progressive lenses also have some limitations and challenges, such as peripheral distortion, adaptation difficulties, and reduced visual fields. Therefore, there is a need for advanced design of progressive lenses that can overcome these drawbacks and enhance the visual performance and comfort of the users.

One of the main needs for the advanced design of progressive lenses is to optimize the optical quality and minimize the aberrations across the entire lens surface. Aberrations are optical defects that cause blurring, ghosting, or halos in the vision. They are mainly caused by the complex geometry and power variation of progressive lenses. To reduce aberrations, various methods have been proposed, such as using aspheric or atoric surfaces, applying free-form technology, or incorporating the wavefront-guided design. These methods aim to improve the optical quality and enlarge the clear vision zones for both distance and near vision.

Another need for advanced design of progressive lenses is to customize the lens parameters according to the individual characteristics and preferences of the users. Different users may have different visual demands, eye movements, head postures, and facial features that affect their adaptation and satisfaction with progressive lenses. Therefore, it is important to consider these factors when designing progressive lenses and adjust the parameters such as addition power, corridor length, fitting height, inset, and decentration. By doing so, the lens design can match the user's visual behaviour and ergonomic needs and provide a more comfortable and natural vision.

A third need for advanced design of progressive lenses is to incorporate new technologies and materials that can enhance the functionality and durability of the lenses. For example, some progressive lenses can incorporate smart features such as photochromic, polarized, or blue-light-blocking properties that can adapt to different light conditions and protect the eyes from harmful radiation. Some progressive lenses can also use materials such as high-index, polycarbonate, or trivex that can make the lenses thinner, lighter, and more resistant to impact or scratches. These technologies and materials can improve the aesthetic and safety aspects of progressive lenses and increase their appeal to users.

In conclusion, progressive lenses are a popular and effective solution for presbyopic patients who need multifocal correction. However, they also have some limitations that can compromise the visual quality and comfort of the users. Therefore, there is a need for advanced design of progressive lenses that can address these issues and provide a better visual experience for the users. Some of the needs for advanced design of progressive lenses are to optimize the optical quality and minimize aberrations, to customize the lens parameters according to individual factors, and to incorporate new technologies and materials that can enhance functionality and durability.

References:
Sheedy JE, Hardy RF. The optics of progressive addition lenses. Optom Vis Sci. 1988;65(3):162-168.
Jalie M. Ophthalmic Lenses & Dispensing. 4th ed. Elsevier; 2018.
Charman WN. Developments in the correction of presbyopia

II: surgical approaches. Ophthalmic Physiol Opt. 2014;34(4):397-426.

Meister DJ, Fisher SW. Progress in the spectacle correction of presbyopia. Part 2: Modern progressive lens technologies. Clin Exp Optom. 2018;101(1):11-22.

ADVANCED DESIGN PROGRESSIVE ADDITION LENSES COME WITH

Advanced design Progressive Addition Lenses (PALs) are a type of multifocal lenses that provide a continuous and smooth transition from distance to near vision, without any visible lines or segments. PALs are designed to meet the visual needs of presbyopic patients, who have difficulty focusing on near objects due to the age-related loss of accommodation of the eye. PALs offer several advantages over conventional bifocal or trifocal lenses, such as a wider field of clear vision, a more comfortable intermediate vision, continuous support to the eye's accommodation, and a more natural perception of space and movement.

Progressive Addition Lenses (PAL) are designed using sophisticated optical software that optimizes the lens surface to minimize unwanted astigmatism and maximize channel width. Unwanted astigmatism is the difference between the actual power of the lens and the prescribed power, which causes blur and distortion in the peripheral areas of the lens. Channel width is the horizontal distance between two points on the lens where the unwanted astigmatism is equal to a certain value, usually 0.5 diopters. A wider channel width means a larger area of clear vision for the wearer.

PALs are also designed asymmetrically, meaning that the right and left lenses have different surface profiles to account for the different eye movements and postures of the wearer. For example, PALs may have a steeper power progression on the nasal side and a flatter power progression on the temporal side, to reduce unwanted astigmatism and increase channel width in the reading zone. PALs may also have different designs for different types of wearers or applications, such as occupational lenses, computer lenses, or sports lenses.

The optical quality and performance of PALs can be described and controlled by various parameters, such as power profile, contour plot, grid plot, and three-dimensional plot. These parameters show how the power of the lens changes across its surface, and how it affects the vision of the wearer. A power profile is a graph that shows the change in power along a vertical meridian of the lens, from distance to near zone. A contour plot is a map that shows the contours of equal power on the lens surface. A grid plot is a map that shows the values of power or unwanted astigmatism on a grid of points on the lens surface. A three-dimensional plot is a graph that shows the power of unwanted astigmatism as a function of horizontal and vertical coordinates on the lens surface.

PALs are manufactured using either cast moulding or free-form surfacing techniques. Cast moulding involves pouring liquid resin into a mould that has the desired surface profile of the lens. Free-form surfacing involves cutting and polishing the lens surface using computer-controlled machines that follow the design data. Free-form surfacing allows more flexibility and customization in producing PALs with complex surface profiles.

PALs are prescribed based on the patient's refractive error, near addition, interpupillary distance, fitting height, frame size and shape, and visual preferences. The fitting height is the vertical distance from the centre of the pupil to the lower edge of the frame, which determines how much of the lens surface is available for distance, intermediate, and near vision. The frame size and shape affect how well the lens design matches the wearer's visual field. The visual preferences of the patient may influence the choice of lens design, such as whether they prefer a wider intermediate zone or a faster near transition.

`PALs are fitted by measuring and marking the fitting cross on each lens, which indicates the position of the distance reference point (DRP) and the fitting point (FP). The DRP is the point on the lens where the prescribed distance power is provided. The FP is the point on the lens where the optical axis of the eye should be aligned when looking straight ahead. The fitting cross should be aligned with the centre of the pupil when fitting PALs to ensure optimal vision.

The following are some scientific journal and book references in APA7 style that provide more information about PALs:

Ang, W., & Sheedy, J.E. (2011). Progressive addition lenses: measurements and rating systems. In B.L. Cole (Ed.), Progressive addition lenses: Achieving patient satisfaction (pp. 1-22). Butterworth-Heinemann.

Jalie, M., & Wray Lyle S. (2002). Ophthalmic lenses & dispensing (3rd ed.). Butterworth-Heinemann.

Sheedy J.E., & Hardy R.F. (1987). Optics of progressive addition lenses: problems and solutions in progressive addition lens design and use. Journal of Optometry, 64(4), 539-546.

Smith G., & Atchison D.A. (1997). The eye and visual optical instruments. Cambridge University Press.

Varilux progressive lenses. (n.d.). Essilor. Retrieved October 17, 2023, from https://www.essilor.com/en/brands/varilux/

MARKETING OF ADVANCED DESIGN PALS

Progressive lenses also pose some challenges for both the optometrist and the patient. The optometrist needs to perform a careful and accurate measurement of the patient's eyes and prescribe the most suitable progressive lens design for their visual needs and preferences. The patient needs to adapt to the progressive lens and learn how to use it properly, which may take some time and practice. Moreover, the patient needs to be aware of the benefits and limitations of progressive lenses and have realistic expectations about their performance.

Therefore, marketing progressive lenses requires a comprehensive and strategic approach that involves educating the patient, providing personalized service, and ensuring customer satisfaction. In this chapter, we will discuss some of the best marketing ways of advanced design of progressive lenses, based on the latest research and industry trends. We will cover the following topics:
- The evolution and innovation of progressive lens design
- The factors that influence the patient's choice and satisfaction with progressive lenses
- The methods and tools for measuring and fitting progressive lenses
- The tips and techniques for training and educating the patient on progressive lens use
- The strategies and tactics for promoting and selling progressive lenses
- The challenges and opportunities for the future of progressive lens marketing

These are some useful information and guidance for optometrists, opticians, and other eye care professionals who want to improve their marketing skills and increase their sales of progressive lenses.

References:
- Benavente-Pérez A, Nagra M, Logan NS. The effect of phenylephrine on the ciliary muscle and accommodation. Ophthalmic Physiol Opt. 2012;32(1):89-98.
- Charman WN. Developments in the correction of presbyopia I: spectacle and contact lenses. Ophthalmic Physiol Opt. 2014;34(1):8-29.
- Sheedy JE, Hardy RF, Hayes JR. Progressive addition lenses--measurements and ratings. Optom Vis Sci. 2006;83(2):146-158.
- Varma R, Richman EA, Ferris FL 3rd, Bressler NM. Use of vision-related quality of life in clinical practice as an outcome variable: an update from the American Academy of Ophthalmology Task Force on Clinical Outcomes Assessment. Ophthalmology. 2019;126(6):855-859.
- Zikos GA, Kang SY, Ciuffreda KJ. Analysis of progressive addition lens fit using an infrared reflection technique. Optom Vis Sci. 2007;84(12):1105-1111.

THE EVOLUTION AND INNOVATION OF PAL DESIGN

The history of progressive lenses dates back to the late 19th century when the first attempts to create a lens with a variable power were made. However, these early prototypes had many drawbacks, such as distortion, aberration, and limited fields of view. The first commercially successful progressive lens was introduced in 1959 by Bernard Maitenaz, a French engineer working for Essilor. Maitenaz's invention, called Varilux, was based on a complex mathematical formula that calculated the optimal surface curvature for each point on the lens. Varilux revolutionized the optical industry and paved the way for further research and development of progressive lens design.

Since then, progressive lenses have undergone many improvements and innovations, both in terms of design and manufacturing. Some of the major milestones in the evolution of progressive lens design are:

In the 1970s, computer-aided design (CAD) and computer-aided manufacturing (CAM) technologies were introduced, allowing for more precise and customized lens production.

In the 1980s, soft design techniques were developed, which reduced the unwanted astigmatism and distortion in the peripheral zones of the lens.

In the 1990s, free-form technology was introduced, which enabled the creation of progressive lenses with complex and asymmetric surface shapes, tailored to the individual wearer's prescription and preferences.

In the 2000s, personalized progressive lenses were developed, which took into account not only the wearer's prescription, but also other factors such as eye anatomy, facial measurements, frame characteristics, and visual behaviour.

In the 2010s, digital progressive lenses were developed, which used advanced algorithms and software to optimize the lens performance for different viewing situations and environments.

The innovation of progressive lens design continues today, with new technologies and materials that aim to enhance the visual comfort and satisfaction of presbyopic patients. Some of the current trends and challenges in progressive lens design are:

The development of smart progressive lenses, which can adapt to the wearer's changing visual needs and preferences, using sensors, actuators, or electronic components.

The integration of progressive lenses with other devices or applications, such as augmented reality (AR), virtual reality (VR), or artificial intelligence (AI), provides new functionalities and experiences for the wearer.

The improvement of progressive lenses for specific purposes or populations, such as sports, driving, children, or low vision.

The evaluation of progressive lenses using objective and subjective methods, such as optical quality measurements, visual acuity tests, or quality of life surveys.

Progressive lenses are one of the most successful and widely used optical solutions for presbyopia correction. They have evolved and innovated over time to meet the diverse and demanding needs of modern presbyopic patients. Progressive lens design is a dynamic and interdisciplinary field that combines science, engineering, art, and psychology. It is expected that progressive lens design will continue to advance and innovate in the future, offering new possibilities and benefits for presbyopic patients and society at large.

References:

- Benard Y., D.A. Atchison & L.N. Thibos (2010). "Optics of Progressive Addition Lenses". In: D.A. Atchison & G. Smith (eds.), Optics of the Human Eye. Elsevier.
- Sheedy J.E., R.A. Hardy & P.A. Hayes (2006). "Progressive Addition Lenses - Measurements and Ratings". In: B. Benjamin (ed.), Borish's Clinical Refraction (2nd ed.). Elsevier.
- Varilux.com (2021). "The Varilux Story". Retrieved from https://www.varilux.com/en/the-varilux-story

THE FACTORS INFLUENCE PATIENT SATISFACTION

The factors that influence the patient's choice and satisfaction with progressive lenses can be divided into three categories: patient-related factors, lens-related factors, and environmental factors. Patient-related factors include the patient's age, refractive error, visual needs, expectations, preferences, personality, and lifestyle. Lens-related factors include the lens design, material, power distribution, addition power, corridor length and width, near zone size and shape, fitting height, decentration, tilt, wrap angle, and coating. Environmental factors include lighting conditions, visual tasks, working distance, posture, head and eye movements, and adaptation period. These factors interact with each other and affect the patient's visual performance and comfort with progressive lenses.

Patient-related factors

The following is a brief overview of each factor and its impact on the patient's choice and satisfaction with progressive lenses:

Age: As the patient ages, the lens of the eye becomes less flexible and loses its ability to accommodate or change focus from far to near. This results in presbyopia, which requires a correction for near vision in addition to distance vision. The degree of presbyopia varies from person to person and depends on the initial refractive error and the amount of accommodation loss. The older the patient, the higher the additional power needed for near vision. However, a higher addition power also means a greater difference between the distance and near zones of the progressive lens, which can cause more distortion and blur in the intermediate zone. Therefore, the patient's age affects the choice of the appropriate addition power and lens design for progressive lenses.

Refractive error: The patient's refractive error is the amount of correction needed for distance vision. It can be classified into three types: myopia (nearsightedness), hyperopia (farsightedness), and astigmatism (irregular curvature of the cornea or lens). The refractive error affects the choice of the base curve and power distribution of the progressive lens. A higher refractive error requires a steeper base curve and a more complex power distribution to minimize aberrations and provide a clear image at all distances. However, a steeper base curve also increases the thickness and weight of the lens, which can affect the cosmetic appearance and comfort of the patient. Therefore, the patient's refractive error affects the balance between optical quality and aesthetic appeal of progressive lenses.

Visual needs: Visual needs refer to the activities and tasks that require different levels of visual acuity and field of view. Patients who perform a lot of near work or computer work may prefer progressive lenses that have wider near and intermediate zones than those who mainly use distance vision. Patients who drive a lot or play sports may need progressive lenses that have minimal distortion and good peripheral vision.

Expectations and preferences: Expectations and preferences are related to the patient's satisfaction with the appearance, performance, and cost of progressive lenses. Patients who expect progressive lenses to provide perfect vision in all situations may be disappointed and dissatisfied with the limitations and compromises of progressive lenses. Patients who prefer a certain design, brand, or material of progressive lenses may be more satisfied with their choice than those who do not have a preference.

Personality and lifestyle: Personality and lifestyle are factors that reflect the patient's attitude, behaviour, and adaptation to progressive lenses. Patients who are optimistic, flexible, and willing to learn may adapt faster and better to progressive lenses than those who are pessimistic, rigid, and resistant to change. Patients who have an active and dynamic lifestyle may need more time and effort to adjust to progressive lenses than those who have a stable and routine lifestyle.

Some references for these factors are:

Sheedy JE, Hardy RF, Hayes JR. Progressive addition lenses--measurements and ratings. Optom Vis Sci. 2006;83(2):75-83.

Woods J, Woods CA, Fonn D. Early symptomatic adaptation to progressive addition lenses. Optom Vis Sci. 1996;73(8):533-9.

Montés-Micó R, Ferrer-Blasco T, Cerviño A. Visual performance with multifocal soft contact lenses: a clinical trial. Ophthalmic Physiol Opt. 2007;27(1):45-9.

Hennessey D, Ito H, Rucker FJ. The effect of personality on subjective satisfaction with spectacles among presbyopes in Japan: a pilot study. Clin Exp Optom. 2010;93(5):329-35.

Lens-related factors

Lens-related factors include the lens design, material, power distribution, addition power, corridor length and width, near zone size and shape, fitting height, decentration, tilt, wrap angle, and coating.

Lens design refers to the optical form and configuration of a lens, such as spherical, aspherical, cylindrical, or toroidal. Lens design affects the image quality, aberrations, field of view, and magnification of a lens. Different types of lens designs are suitable for different applications and purposes.

Material refers to the substance that a lens is made of, such as glass, plastic, or polymer. Material affects the refractive index, dispersion, transmission, absorption, weight, durability, and cost of a lens. Different types of materials have different optical properties and trade-offs.

Power distribution refers to the way that the optical power of a lens varies across its surface. Power distribution affects the focal length, astigmatism, distortion, and depth of field of a lens. Different types of power distributions are used for different vision corrections and enhancements.

Addition power refers to the difference in optical power between the distance and near portions of a multifocal lens. Addition power affects the near vision acuity, accommodation, convergence, and eye strain of a wearer. Different levels of additional power are prescribed for different presbyopic conditions.

Corridor length and width refer to the dimensions of the progressive zone of a multifocal lens that connects the distance and near portions. Corridor length and width affect the smoothness, clarity, and comfort of the transition between different viewing distances. Different sizes of corridors are designed for different frame shapes and wearer preferences.

Near zone size and shape refer to the area of a multifocal lens that provides near vision correction. Near zone size and shape affect the reading performance, visual field, and peripheral vision of a wearer. Different shapes and sizes of near zones are optimized for different reading tasks and environments.

Fitting height refers to the vertical distance from the centre of the pupil to the lower edge of the frame when a wearer is looking straight ahead. Fitting height affects the position and alignment of the lens of the eye. Different fitting heights are required for different types of multifocal lenses and frame styles.

Decentration refers to the horizontal displacement of the optical centre of a lens from the centre of the pupil when a wearer is looking straight ahead. Decentration affects the prismatic effect, binocular vision, and visual comfort of a wearer. Different amounts of decentration are needed for different prescriptions and pupillary distances.

Tilt refers to the angle between the optical axis of a lens and the line perpendicular to the plane of the frame when a wearer is looking straight ahead. Tilt affects the effective power, aberrations, and image quality of a lens. Different angles of tilt are induced by different frame shapes and fitting styles.

Wrap angle refers to the angle between the plane of a lens and the plane perpendicular to the line connecting the temples of a frame when a wearer is looking straight ahead. Wrap angle affects the peripheral vision, distortion, and magnification of a lens. Different angles of wrap are associated with different frame designs and curvatures.

Coating refers to the thin layer or layers of material that are applied to the surface of a lens to modify its optical properties or protect it from damage. Coating affects the reflection, transmission, absorption, polarization, anti-glare, scratch-resistance, water-repellence, and appearance of a lens. Different types of coatings are available for different purposes and preferences.

References:

Optical Lens Design Forms: An Ultimate Guide to the types of Lens Design (https://www.pencilofrays.com/lens-design-forms/)

Tips for Designing Manufacturable Lenses and Assemblies - Edmund Optics (https://www.edmundoptics.com/knowledge-center/application-notes/optics/tips-for-designing-manufacturable-lenses-and-assemblies/)

Environmental factors

Environmental factors include lighting conditions, visual tasks, working distance, posture, head and eye movements, and adaptation period. These factors can affect the quality and comfort of vision, as well as the risk of developing eye disorders.

Lighting conditions refer to the intensity, colour, direction, and contrast of light sources in the environment. Lighting conditions can influence visual acuity, colour perception, glare sensitivity, and visual fatigue. For example, low light levels can reduce visual acuity and colour discrimination, while high light levels can cause glare and discomfort. Optimal lighting conditions depend on the type and duration of the visual task, as well as the individual preferences and needs of the viewer.

Visual tasks are activities that require visual attention and processing, such as reading, writing, driving, or using a computer. Visual tasks vary in their complexity, size, distance, and duration. Visual tasks can affect the demand and strain on the visual system, as well as the eye movements and accommodation required to perform them. For example, complex or small visual tasks can increase the need for convergence and accommodation, while long or continuous visual tasks can cause eye fatigue and dryness. Optimal visual tasks should be appropriate for the viewer's age, visual abilities, and goals.

Working distance is the distance between the eyes and the object of interest. The working distance can affect the amount of accommodation and convergence needed to focus on the object, as well as the field of view and depth perception available. For example, short working distances can increase the demand on the near vision system, while long working distances can reduce the amount of detail and context perceived. Optimal working distances should be comfortable and adjustable for the viewer and the task.

Posture is the position and alignment of the body and its parts. Posture can affect the blood circulation, muscle tension, and breathing patterns of the viewer, as well as the angle and direction of gaze. For example, poor posture can cause neck and back pain, headaches, and reduced oxygen intake, while good posture can enhance alertness, comfort, and performance. Optimal posture should be relaxed, balanced, and supported for the viewer and the task.

Head and eye movements are the voluntary or involuntary motions of the head and eyes in response to stimuli or tasks. Head and eye movements can affect the stability and coordination of vision, as well as the vestibular system and balance. For example, excessive or rapid head and eye movements can cause dizziness, nausea, and blurred vision, while insufficient or slow head and eye movements can cause stiffness, fatigue, or reduced attention. Optimal head and eye movements should be smooth, accurate, and efficient for the viewer and the task.

Adaptation period is the time required for the eyes to adjust to changes in lighting conditions or viewing distances. Adaptation period can affect the speed and quality of vision recovery after exposure to different environments or tasks. For example, long adaptation periods can cause temporary visual impairment or discomfort after switching from bright to dark environments or from near to far objects. Short adaptation periods can enhance visual flexibility and resilience in changing situations. Optimal adaptation periods depend on the individual characteristics and experiences of the viewer.

Environmental factors play an important role in maintaining eye health and vision quality. By understanding how these factors affect vision, one can take preventive measures to protect their eyes from potential harm or discomfort.

References:
Environmental Effects on Color Vision | SpringerLink
Environmental factors affecting vision - SlideShare.
Environmental factors and eye health: Protecting your vision in a changing world.

MEASURING AND FITTING PROGRESSIVE LENSES

*The methods and tools for measuring
and fitting progressive lenses*

The methods and tools for measuring and fitting progressive lenses are essential for ensuring optimal visual performance and comfort for presbyopic patients. Progressive lenses provide a smooth transition from distance to near vision, without the need for bifocal lines or segment boundaries. However, they also require careful fitting and adjustment to match the patient's needs and preferences.

*Some of the steps involved
in measuring and fitting
progressive lenses are*

Selecting the appropriate frame size, shape, and style for the patient's facial features, prescription, and lifestyle. The frame should have enough vertical depth to accommodate the full range of the progressive lens and should be stable and comfortable on the patient's face.

Pre-adjusting the frame to fit the patient's face before taking any measurements. The frame should be aligned with the patient's eyes, ears, and nose, and should have adequate pantoscopic tilt, vertex distance, and wrap angle.

Measuring the fitting heights for each eye, which is the distance from the lower rim of the frame to the centre of the pupil. The fitting heights determine where the fitting cross or reference point (FRP) of the progressive lens will be located on the lens. The FRP is the point that should coincide with the patient's pupil when looking straight ahead. The fitting heights should be marked on the demo lenses or a lensometer chart.

Measuring the distance pupillary distance (PDs) for each eye, which is the distance from the centre of the nose to the centre of the pupil. The distance PDs determine where the optical centres of the lenses will be located on the lens. The optical centres should be aligned with the patient's pupils when looking at a distant object. The distance PDs can be measured using a PD ruler, a corneal reflex pupillometer, or a digital measuring device.

Verifying the cut-out of the lenses, which is the minimum blank size required to fit the lenses into the frame without compromising the optical quality or design of the progressive lens. The cut-out can be checked using a layout chart or a digital tracing device.

Taking free-form measurements (if necessary), which are additional parameters that can be used to customize the progressive lens design for each patient. These include near PDs, near working distance, pantoscopic tilt, vertex distance, wrap angle, back vertex distance, and frame dimensions. These measurements can be taken using a digital measuring device or a manual method.

The tools used for measuring and fitting progressive lenses include:
- A PD ruler or a corneal reflex pupillometer for measuring distance PDs
- A pen light or a pupilometer for measuring fitting heights

- A layout chart or a digital tracing device for verifying cut-out
- A digital measuring device or a manual method for taking free-form measurements
- A lensometer or a verification chart for verifying lens properties

The sources used for generating this text are:

Fitting and Dispensing Progressive Lenses Troubleshooting Fitting Issues - EssilorPRO https://www.essilorpro.com/content/dam/essilor-pro/product-resources/varilux/LVAR201326_Varilux_Fitting_N_Dispensing_Guide_LR.pdf

Progressive Lenses Fitting Guide | Essilor Academy https://www.essiloracademy.eu/en/publications-progressive-lenses-fitting-guide

VARILUX FITTING GUIDE - Essilor Academy https://www.essiloracademy.eu/pdf_server.php?file=/sites/default/files/Guide_US.pdf

Progressive Lens Dispensing - opticampus. opti.vision http://opticampus.opti.vision/files/progressive_lens_dispensing.pdf

TRAINING THE PATIENT ON PROGRESSIVE LENS USE

Progressive lenses are designed using state-of-the-art optical technology, and when adjusted to the individual's specific needs, they provide great wearer satisfaction. However, some patients may need some training and education on how to use progressive lenses effectively and comfortably. Here are some tips and techniques for doing so:

Explain the benefits of progressive lenses to the patient about their lifestyle, needs and preferences. For example, if the patient likes to read books, watch TV and drive, you can tell them how progressive lenses will eliminate the need for switching between different pairs of glasses for each activity. You can also use positive testimonials from other patients or your own experience to illustrate the advantages of progressive lenses.

Demonstrate how to use progressive lenses properly by showing the patient how to move their eyes and head when looking at different distances. For example, you can ask the patient to look at a near object, such as a book or a smartphone, through the lower part of the lens, then look at a far object, such as a sign or a clock, through the upper part of the lens. You can also point out the intermediate zone of the lens, which is useful for viewing objects at arm's length, such as a computer screen or a dashboard.

Help the patient adjust to progressive lenses gradually by

advising them to wear them as much as possible during the first few days or weeks. You can also suggest some exercises to help them get used to the different zones of the lens, such as reading a newspaper from top to bottom, scanning a room from left to right, or looking at objects at various distances. You can also reassure the patient that any initial discomfort or distortion will subside as their eyes and brain adapt to the new lenses.

Choose the best lens design for the patient based on their prescription, frame size, pupil position, eye dominance, binocular vision and visual habits. You can use a lifestyle questionnaire or checklist to gather this information from the patient or ask them directly about their work, activities and hobbies. You can also use precise measurements and fitting tools to ensure that the lens is aligned correctly with the patient's eyes.

Follow up with the patient after dispensing the progressive lenses to check their satisfaction, comfort and vision quality. You can ask them for feedback on how they are using the lenses, what they like or dislike about them, and if they have any questions or concerns. You can also make any necessary adjustments or modifications to the lenses or frames if needed.

By following these tips and techniques, you can help your patient enjoy the benefits of progressive lenses and improve their quality of life.

References:
https://www.unitylenses.com/blog/presenting-progressive-lens-
    benefits-to-patients
https://www.zeiss.com/vision-care/us/eye-health-and-care/
    driving-mobility/tips-for-better-wearing-comfort-of-
    progressive-lenses.html
https://www.reviewofoptometry.com/article/professional-
    pearls-for-fitting-pals

CHALLENGES AND OPPORTUNITIES FOR THE FUTURE

One of the main strategies for promoting and selling progressive lenses is to educate the customers about the benefits and advantages of these lenses over traditional bifocals or trifocals. Progressive lenses offer a more natural and comfortable visual experience, as they allow the users to smoothly transition from one focal point to another, without any abrupt changes or distortions. Progressive lenses also eliminate the need for multiple pairs of glasses or switching between glasses and contact lenses, which can be inconvenient and costly. Moreover, progressive lenses have a more aesthetic appeal, as they do not reveal the age or presbyopia status of the wearer.

Another strategy is to differentiate the progressive lenses from the competitors by highlighting the unique features and technologies of each brand and product. For example, ZEISS Progressive lenses are based on ZEISS SmartView Technology, which optimises the lens design according to the customer's lifestyle, visual behaviour, frame choice and facial anatomy. ZEISS also offers a range of progressive lens options, such as ZEISS Progressive SmartLife Pure, Plus, Superb and Individual 3, to suit different customer needs and preferences (ZEISS, n.d.). Similarly, Essilor Progressive lenses, such as Varilux, are supported by Essilor W.A.V.E Technology 2™, which reduces aberrations and enhances contrast and sharpness in all light conditions. Essilor also provides a variety of progressive lens solutions, such as Varilux X series™, Varilux E series™ and Varilux Physio 3.0™, to cater to different customer expectations and lifestyles (Essilor India, n.d.).

A third strategy Is to use effective marketing tools and channels to communicate the value proposition and brand identity of the progressive lenses to the target audience. This can include using online platforms, such as websites, social media, blogs and videos, to showcase the product features, testimonials, reviews and demonstrations of the progressive lenses. For instance, progressive-glasses.com is a blog that provides information, tips and advice on progressive lenses from various brands, such as ZEISS, Essilor, Rodenstock and Hoya. The blog also features images and videos that illustrate the differences between progressive lenses and other types of lenses (Progressive Glasses Brands, n.d.). Additionally, offline methods, such as brochures, flyers, posters and banners, can be used to display the product benefits, logos and engravings of the progressive lenses in eye care stores or clinics. These can help to increase brand awareness and recognition among potential customers (What Are the Markings on My Progressive Lenses? n.d.).

References:

Essilor India. (n.d.). Progressive Lenses for Clear Vision at All Distance | Essilor India. Retrieved October 18, 2023 from https://www.essilorindia.com/products/progressive-lenses

Progressive Glasses Brands. (n.d.). Progressive Glasses Brands. Retrieved October 18, 2023 from https://progressive-glasses.com/progressive-glasses-brands/

What Are the Markings on My Progressive Lenses? (n.d.). What Are the Markings on My Progressive Lenses? Retrieved October 18, 2023, from https://progressive-glasses.com/what-are-the-markings-on-my-progressive-lenses/

ZEISS. (n.d.). ZEISS Progressive lenses. Retrieved October 18, 2023, from https://www.zeiss.co.in/vision-care/eye-care-professionals/lenses/lens-type/progressive-lenses.html

The challenges and opportunities for the future of progressive lens marketing

One of the main challenges for progressive lens marketing is the high cost and complexity of the product, which may deter some potential customers from trying or buying it. Progressive lenses require precise measurements, fitting, and adaptation by trained professionals, and they are usually more expensive than single-vision or bifocal lenses. Moreover, some users may experience initial discomfort, distortion, or dizziness when wearing progressive lenses, especially if they are not properly fitted or adjusted. Therefore, progressive lens marketing needs to educate consumers about the benefits and features of progressive lenses, as well as address their possible concerns and objections.

Another challenge for progressive lens marketing is the increasing competition from online retailers and low-cost alternatives, such as ready-made reading glasses or contact lenses. Online retailers can offer lower prices and convenience for customers who already have a prescription and know their preferences. However, they may not provide the same level of quality, accuracy, or service as offline opticians or optical shops. Low-cost alternatives, such as ready-made reading glasses or contact lenses, may appeal to customers who only need occasional or temporary correction for near vision. However, they may not provide the optimal solution for customers who need continuous or comprehensive vision correction for different distances. Therefore, progressive lens marketing needs to differentiate its product from online retailers and low-cost alternatives, by emphasizing its value proposition, quality, and customization.

One of the main opportunities for progressive lens marketing is the growing demand and potential market for presbyopia correction, especially among the ageing population and the digital generation. Presbyopia affects more than one billion people worldwide, and it is expected to increase as the population ages. Moreover, the digital generation, who spend long hours using computers, smartphones, and other devices, may experience early onset or worsening of presbyopia symptoms, such as eye strain, headaches, or blurred vision. Therefore, progressive lens marketing needs to target these segments with relevant messages and offers that appeal to their needs and lifestyles.

Another opportunity for progressive lens marketing is the innovation and development of new technologies and designs that enhance the performance and appeal of progressive lenses. For example, some progressive lenses incorporate digital surfacing technology that allows for more precise and customized lens design and fabrication. Some progressive lenses also feature advanced coatings or materials that reduce glare, reflections, or scratches, and improve contrast, clarity, or durability. Moreover, some progressive lenses offer various options for colours, shapes, or styles that suit different preferences and occasions. Therefore, progressive lens marketing needs to showcase these innovations and developments that improve the customer experience and satisfaction with progressive lenses.

In conclusion, progressive lens marketing faces several challenges and opportunities for the future in a dynamic and competitive environment. Progressive lens marketing needs to adopt effective strategies and tactics that address the customer pain points and highlight the product benefits and advantages. Progressive lens marketing also needs to leverage the market trends and opportunities that create more demand and interest for progressive lenses among different segments.

References:

American Optometric Association. (n.d.). Presbyopia. Retrieved from https://www.aoa.org/patients-and-public/eye-and-vision-problems/glossary-of-eye-and-vision-conditions/presbyopia

Essilor. (n.d.). What are progressive lenses? Retrieved from https://www.essilor.com/en/vision-correction/presbyopia/progressive-lenses/

Vision Service Plan. (n.d.). Progressive Lenses: Are They Right for You? Retrieved from https://www.vsp.com/progressive-lenses.html

OTHER MARKETING WAYS OF ADVANCED DESIGN PALS

One of the challenges of marketing progressive lenses is to educate consumers about their benefits and advantages over other types of lenses and to overcome some of the common misconceptions and barriers that may prevent them from choosing progressive lenses. Some of the marketing strategies that can be used to promote progressive lenses are:

Creating awareness campaigns that highlight the features and benefits of progressive lenses, such as improved visual comfort, convenience, aesthetics, and quality of life. These campaigns can use various media channels, such as print, online, social media, radio, television, or outdoor advertising, to reach the target audience and convey the message effectively.

Providing testimonials and endorsements from satisfied customers, celebrities, influencers, or experts who use progressive lenses and can share their positive experiences and outcomes. These testimonials can be featured on the website, social media pages, brochures, or videos of the progressive lens brand or retailer, and can help to build trust and credibility among potential customers.

Offering free trials or discounts for progressive lenses to encourage customers to try them out and experience the difference for themselves. This can help to overcome some of the initial resistance or hesitation that customers may have about switching to progressive lenses, especially if they are used to wearing bifocal or trifocal lenses. Free trials or discounts can also create a sense of urgency and incentive for customers to make a purchase decision.

Providing professional guidance and support for customers who are interested in progressive lenses, such as eye exams, fitting, adjustment, follow-up, and after-sales service. This can help to ensure that customers are satisfied with their progressive lenses and can use them comfortably and effectively. Professional guidance and support can also help to address any questions or concerns that customers may have about progressive lenses, such as adaptation period, cost, quality, or warranty.

Developing loyalty programs or referral schemes that reward customers who buy progressive lenses or recommend them to others. This can help to retain existing customers and attract new ones, as well as create a positive word-of-mouth effect. Loyalty programs or referral schemes can offer various incentives, such as points, vouchers, gifts, or discounts, for customers who buy progressive lenses or refer their friends or family members to do so.

These are some of the marketing ways that can be used to promote the advanced design of progressive lenses and increase their market share and customer satisfaction. Progressive lenses are a valuable solution for presbyopic customers who want to enjoy clear and comfortable vision at all distances and in all situations.

References:
American Optometric Association. (2020). Presbyopia. Retrieved from https://www.aoa.org/healthy-eyes/eye-and-vision-conditions/presbyopia
Essilor. (2020). What are progressive lenses? Retrieved from https://www.essilor.co.uk/progressive-lenses/what-are-

progressive-lenses

Vision Service Plan. (2020). Progressive Lenses: Are They Right for You? Retrieved from https://www.vsp.com/progressive-lenses.html

What are the advanced design PALs available in the market?

Progressive addition lenses (PALs) are a type of multifocal lens that provide a smooth transition of power from distance to near vision, without any visible lines or segments. PALs are designed to correct presbyopia, a condition that affects most people over the age of 40, causing difficulty in focusing on near objects. PALs are also known as varifocal, no-line, or seamless bifocal lenses.

There are many different designs of PALs available in the market, each with its advantages and disadvantages. Some of the factors that influence the design of PALs are:

- The shape and size of the lens
- The distribution and progression of power across the lens
- The amount and location of astigmatism and distortion in the lens
- The width and length of the corridor (the area of gradual power change)
- The position and shape of the near and intermediate zones
- The personalization and customization of the lens for each wearer

AVAILABLE ADVANCED DESIGN PALS IN THE MARKET

Freeform PALs: These are PALs that are digitally customized for each wearer, using computer-controlled machines to cut and polish the complex surfaces of the lens. Freeform PALs can offer more precise and accurate vision correction, as well as wider fields of view and reduced aberrations. Freeform PALs can also be tailored to specific visual needs and preferences, such as occupational or lifestyle demands.

Aspheric PALs: These are PALs that have a flatter and thinner profile than conventional spherical lenses, reducing the magnification and minification effects that can distort the appearance of the eyes and face. Aspheric PALs can also improve peripheral vision and reduce edge blur, especially for high prescriptions.

Atoric PALs: These are PALs that have different curvatures on the front and back surfaces of the lens, creating a toric shape that can correct astigmatism more effectively. Atoric PALs can also reduce unwanted astigmatism and distortion in the lens, improving visual quality and comfort.

Trifocal PALs: These are PALs that have three distinct zones of power: distance, intermediate, and near. Trifocal PALs can provide clearer and sharper vision for intermediate tasks, such as computer work or reading labels, compared to conventional bifocal or progressive lenses. Trifocal PALs can also reduce the need for head movements or postural changes when switching between different viewing distances.

Some scientific journal and book references for further reading on advanced design PALs are:

Mukhopadhyay, D. (2019). Advanced designs of progressive addition lenses over conventional. Retrieved from https://www.researchgate.net/profile/Debapriya-Mukhopadhyay/publication/335812629_Advance_designs_of_progressive_addition_lenses_over_conventional/links/5d7c7446a6fdcc2f0f6dd421/Advance-designs-of-progressive-addition-lenses-over-conventional.pdf

Sheedy, J. E., & Shaw-McMinn, P. G. (2015). Prescribing multifocal lenses. In B. M. Grosvenor & R. A. Flom (Eds.), Primary care optometry (6th ed., pp. 347-377). Elsevier.

Smith III, G., & Atchison, D. A. (2018). Progressive addition lenses: Design considerations. In G. Smith III & D. A. Atchison (Eds.), Optics of the human eye (2nd ed., pp. 245-260). Elsevier.

What are the brands of advanced design PALs available in the market?

Progressive addition lenses (PALs) are a type of multifocal lenses that provide a smooth transition of power from distance to near vision, without any visible lines or segments. PALs are designed to correct presbyopia, a condition that affects most people over the age of 40, causing difficulty in focusing on near objects.

There are many brands of advanced-design PALs available in the market, each with different features and benefits. Some of the factors that influence the choice of PALs are the lens material, the lens design, the lens coating, the lens fitting, and the wearer's lifestyle and preferences.

According to a research paper by Debapriya Mukhopadhyay, some of the advanced design PALs available in the market are:

Varilux by Essilor: Varilux is one of the most popular and widely used brands of PALs, with a range of products for different needs and preferences. Some of the Varilux products are the Varilux X series, Varilux Physio 3.0, Varilux Comfort 3.0, Varilux E series, Varilux Liberty 3.0, and Varilux Road Pilot.

Zeiss by Carl Zeiss Vision: Zeiss is another leading brand of PALs, offering high-quality lenses with innovative technologies and features. Some of the Zeiss products are Zeiss Individual 2, Zeiss Precision Plus, Zeiss Precision Superb, Zeiss Precision Pure, Zeiss DriveSafe, and Zeiss Officelens.

Hoya by Hoya Vision Care: Hoya is a global manufacturer of optical products, including PALs. Some of the Hoya products are Hoya Lifestyle 3, Hoya Sync 3, Hoya MyStyle V+, Hoya Workstyle V +, Hoya ID MyStyle 2, and Hoya ID Workstyle.

Shamir by Shamir Optical Industry: Shamir is a specialized provider of progressive lenses, with a focus on customized solutions and advanced technologies. Some of the Shamir products are Shamir Autograph Intelligence, Shamir Autograph III, Shamir Spectrum+, Shamir Relax, Shamir WorkSpace, and Shamir Computer.

Rodenstock by Rodenstock GmbH: Rodenstock is a German company that produces high-quality lenses and frames. Some of the Rodenstock products are Rodenstock Impression FreeSign 3, Rodenstock Multigressiv MyLife 2, Rodenstock Progressiv PureLife Free 2, Rodenstock Perfection FreeLife 2, and Rodenstock Ergo NearVision.

These are some examples of the progressive lens brands and products available globally as of 2023. However, there may be variations in availability and pricing depending on the country and region. For more details on the technical specifications and features of each product, please refer to the official websites or brochures of the respective brands.

Varilux by Essilor: Varilux is one of the most popular and widely used brands of PALs, with a range of products for different needs and preferences. Some of the Varilux products are the Varilux X series, Varilux Physio 3.0, Varilux Comfort 3.0, Varilux E series, Varilux Liberty 3.0, and Varilux Road Pilot.

SOME SIGNIFICANT PRODUCTS PORTFOLIO

Essilor

Varilux X series: This is the newest and most innovative Varilux lens design available. It features Xtend Technology, a revolutionary new design calculation that significantly extends the area of sharp vision within arm's reach, so patients no longer have to move their heads to find the right spot. It also uses Nanoptix Technology to reduce the off-balance feeling and W.A.V.E Technology 2 to provide sharper vision even in low light. It is available in three options: X Design, X Fit, and X 4D. The X Fit and X 4D lenses are personalized with the patient's near-vision behaviour and head-eye ratio.

Varilux Physio 3.0: This lens design provides smooth transitions from distance to near, with sharp vision at any distance. It uses W.A.V.E Technology 2 to enhance contrast sensitivity and reduce higher-order aberrations. It also uses Binocular Booster Technology to optimize the prescriptions for both eyes, resulting in better binocular vision. It is available in two options: Physio W3+ and Physio DRx.

Varilux Comfort 3.0: This lens design offers a large reading area and easy adaptation for presbyopic patients. It uses Dual Optix Technology to digitally optimize both surfaces of the lens, resulting in improved visual quality and wider fields of vision. It is available in three options: Comfort W2+, Comfort W2+ Fit, and Comfort DRx.

Varilux E series: This lens design is based on the Varilux Comfort 3.0 design but with enhanced features such as Eye Protect System, which filters harmful blue light and UV rays, and Crizal Sapphire UV coating, which reduces reflections and glare.

Varilux Liberty 3.0: This lens design is an entry-level progressive lens that provides clear vision at all distances. It uses Balanced View Control Technology to minimize distortions and maximize visual comfort.

Varilux Road Pilot: This lens design is specially designed for drivers, providing wide fields of vision for distance and intermediate zones, as well as optimal clarity in low-light conditions. It uses Road Brightening Technology to enhance contrast and colour perception on the road.

References:

Essilor. (n.d.). Varilux Progressive Lenses | Essilor. Retrieved October 17, 2023, from https://www.essilorusa.com/products/varilux

EssilorPRO. (n.d.). Varilux XR series | EssilorPRO. Retrieved October 17, 2023, from https://www.essilorpro.com/resources/varilux/varilux-xr-series

Essilor. (n.d.). Varilux Progressive Lens Technology | Essilor. Retrieved October 17, 2023, from https://www.essilorusa.com/products/varilux/progressive-lens-technology

Essilor. (n.d.). Varilux | Vision excellence from near to far - Essilor. Retrieved October 17, 2023, from https://www.essilor.com/uk-en/products/varilux/

HOYA

Hoya by Hoya Vision Care: Hoya is a global manufacturer

of optical products, including progressive addition lenses (PALs). Some of the Hoya products are:

Hoya Lifestyle 3: Advanced lenses tuned to your patient's lifestyle. They offer clear vision at all distances and a seamless transition between near, intermediate, and far zones. They also have Binocular Harmonization Technology, which ensures that the right and left lenses are individually optimized for each eye.

Hoya Sync 3: Single vision lenses designed to reduce digital eye strain. They have a slight boost in power at the bottom of the lens to help the eyes focus more easily on digital screens. They also have BlueControl coating, which filters out harmful blue light emitted by digital devices.

Hoya MyStyle V+: Individualized progressive lenses for constant focus. They are customized based on the patient's personal preferences, lifestyle, and visual behaviour. They use patented technologies such as iD FreeForm Design Technology, Integrated Double Surface Design, and Balanced View Control to provide sharp and stable vision in all directions and distances.

Hoya Workstyle V+: Occupational lenses for near and intermediate vision. They are ideal for people who spend a lot of time on visual tasks at close or intermediate distances, such as reading, writing, or working on a computer. They have three designs: Close, Screen, and Space, which cater to different working distances and visual needs.

Hoya ID MyStyle 2: Personalized progressive lenses for natural vision. They are based on the patient's prescription, frame choice, wearing parameters, and visual behaviour. They use iD FreeForm Design Technology to create a unique lens surface for each eye, resulting in smooth transitions and minimal distortions.

Hoya ID Workstyle: Progressive lenses for specific work environments. They are designed to provide clear and comfortable vision for near and intermediate tasks, such as office work, hobbies, or sports. They have two designs: Indoor and Outdoor, which offer different levels of distance vision and field of view.

References:
Vision Products | Hoya Vision Care. (n.d.). Retrieved October 17, 2023, from https://www.hoyavision.com/in/vision-products/progressive-lenses/hoyalux-id-lifestyle-3/
Vision Products | Hoya Vision Care. (n.d.). Retrieved October 17, 2023, from https://www.hoyavision.com/in/vision-products/single-vision-lenses/sync-iii/
Vision Products | Hoya Vision Care. (n.d.). Retrieved October 17, 2023, from https://www.hoyavision.com/in/vision-products/progressive-lenses/hoyalux-id-mystyle-v/
Vision Products | Hoya Vision Care. (n.d.). Retrieved October 17, 2023, from https://www.hoyavision.com/in/vision-products/occupational-lenses/hoyalux-id-workstyle-v/
Vision Products | Hoya Vision Care. (n.d.). Retrieved October 17, 2023, from https://www.hoyavision.com/in/vision-products/progressive-lenses/hoyalux-id-mystyle-2/
Vision Products | Hoya Vision Care. (n.d.). Retrieved October 17, 2023, from https://www.hoyavision.com/in/vision-products/progressive-lenses/hoyalux-id-workstyle/

Shamir Optical Industry

Shamir Optical Industry is a leading innovator in ophthalmic lens technologies, offering customized solutions and advanced products for various vision needs. Some of the Shamir products are:

Shamir Autograph Intelligence: A progressive lens that adapts to the wearer's visual behaviour and preferences, using artificial intelligence and Eye-Point Technology III™. It provides optimal vision for every distance and activity, with smooth transitions and minimal distortions (Shamir, n.d.-a).

Shamir Autograph III: A progressive lens that balances the wearer's visual needs and posture, using Natural Posture™ and IntelliCorridor™ technologies. It ensures clear vision in all zones, with reduced eye fatigue and head movements (Shamir, n.d.-b).

Shamir Spectrum+: A progressive lens that offers a wide range of design options and customization, using Continuous Design Technology™. It delivers high visual performance and comfort, with enhanced near vision and intermediate vision (Shamir, n.d.-c).

Shamir Relax: A single vision lens that reduces eye strain and fatigue caused by digital devices, using As-Worn Quadro™ technology. It provides a slight boost of power in the lower part of the lens, helping the eye muscles relax and focus more easily (Shamir, n.d.-d).

Shamir WorkSpace: An occupational lens that is designed for near and intermediate tasks, such as working on a computer or reading. It uses Eye-Point Technology AI™ and Visual AI Engine™ to create a personalized lens that matches the wearer's work environment and visual needs (Shamir, n.d.-e).

Shamir Computer: An occupational lens that is designed for near tasks only, such as reading or sewing. It uses Eye-Point Technology AI™ and Visual AI Engine™ to create a personalized lens that provides a wide field of view and clear vision at close distances (Shamir, n.d.-f).

References

Shamir. (n.d.-a). Shamir Autograph Intelligence™. Retrieved October 17, 2023, from https://shamir.com/in/lenses/progressive-lenses/shamir-autograph-intelligence/

Shamir. (n.d.-b). Shamir Autograph III™. Retrieved October 17, 2023, from https://shamir.com/in/lenses/progressive-lenses/shamir-autograph-iii/

Shamir. (n.d.-c). Shamir Spectrum+™. Retrieved October 17, 2023, from https://shamir.com/in/lenses/progressive-lenses/shamir-spectrum/

Shamir. (n.d.-d). Shamir Relax™. Retrieved October 17, 2023, from https://shamir.com/in/lenses/single-vision-lenses/shamir-relax/

Shamir. (n.d.-e). Shamir WorkSpace™. Retrieved October 17, 2023, from https://shamir.com/in/lenses/occupational-lenses/shamir-workspace/

Shamir. (n.d.-f). Shamir Computer™. Retrieved October 17, 2023, from https://shamir.com/in/lenses/occupational-lenses/shamir-computer/

Rodenstock

Rodenstock by Rodenstock GmbH: Rodenstock is a German company that produces high-quality lenses and frames. Some of the Rodenstock products are:

Rodenstock Impression FreeSign 3: These are individual progressive lenses that offer a wide field of vision and smooth transitions. They are customized to the wearer's parameters, such as pupil distance, near working distance, and frame shape. They also have a patented Eye Lens Technology that optimizes the lens surface for each eye.

Rodenstock Multigressiv MyLife 2: These are progressive

lenses that adapt to the wearer's lifestyle and visual needs. They have four different design options: Expert, Allround, Active, and Near. They also have a Solitaire Protect Balance 2 coating that reduces blue light exposure and enhances contrast.

Rodenstock Progressiv PureLife Free 2: These are eco-friendly progressive lenses that are made of organic materials and have a reduced carbon footprint. They offer natural vision and high contrast in all light conditions. They also have a Solitaire Protect Plus 2 coating that protects against scratches, dirt, and water.

Rodenstock Perfection FreeLife 2: These are biometric progressive lenses that are based on the individual biometry of each eye. They measure the shape and size of each eye and use thousands of data points to produce individualized lenses. They offer the sharpest vision at every distance and in every situation.

Rodenstock Ergo NearVision: These are near-vision lenses that are designed for digital device users. They provide clear and comfortable vision for reading, working on the computer, or using a smartphone. They also have a Solitaire Protect Balance coating that reduces eye strain and fatigue caused by blue light.

References:
Rodenstock Impression FreeSign 3 (n.d.). Retrieved from https://www.rodenstock.com/com/en/progressive-lenses/impression-freesign-3.html
Rodenstock Multigressiv MyLife 2 (n.d.). Retrieved from https://www.rodenstock.com/com/en/progressive-lenses/multigressiv-mylife-2.html
Rodenstock Progressiv PureLife Free 2 (n.d.). Retrieved from https://www.rodenstock.com/com/en/progressive-lenses/progressiv-purelife-free-2.html
Rodenstock Perfection FreeLife 2 (n.d.). Retrieved from https://www.rodenstock.com/com/en/biometric-intelligent-

glasses/perfection-freelife-2.html

Rodenstock Ergo NearVision (n.d.). Retrieved from https://www.rodenstock.com/com/en/near-vision-lenses/ergo-nearvision.html

Tokai

Tokai Progressive lenses are a revolutionary type of eyeglass lenses that use neuroscience technology to reduce eye strain and provide smoother and clearer vision. Tokai Progressive lenses are available in two types: Neuro Select and Neuro Resonas. Neuro Select lenses are designed in collaboration with neuroscientists to measure the brain wave responses to comfort and create a bespoke progressive lens design for each wearer. Neuro Resonas lenses are designed with both the front and back surface of the lens being a progressive design and an additional combination with the use of an aspheric lens. This allows for a wider and clearer view area, as well as lighter and thinner lenses. Tokai Progressive lenses are manufactured in Japan with high-quality materials and processes and offer UV protection, high transparency, scratch resistance, and a one-year warranty. Tokai Progressive lenses are suitable for active and outdoorsy people who cannot compromise on their vision quality and comfort.

Tokai Optical is a leading lens manufacturer that uses neuroscience to create bespoke progressive lens designs. Tokai has developed four main neuro technologies that add a level of personalization to the lens design: N-LINK SYSTEM, MYTUNE ENGINE, I LOCATION REMIX & SUPER FLEXIBLE INSET. Two of the products that use these technologies are Neuro Select and Neuro Resonas.

Neuro Select is a high-specification progressive lens that

exploits cutting-edge neuroscience and is selected by the brain, according to the person and their lifestyle. Neuro Select uses the N-LINK SYSTEM, which is a special type of eye test that measures the stress and discomfort of the brain while wearing progressive lenses. The measuring and analysis of brain waves have led to the development of revolutionary progressive lens designs that are easy to adapt to and that reduce the amount of discomfort experienced by the brain. Neuro Select also uses the MYTUNE ENGINE, which is a neurotechnology that adjusts the design parameters based on the wearer's age, prescription, frame size, pupil distance, and visual habits. Neuro Select offers a wide range of options for different activities and lifestyles, such as reading, driving, sports, digital devices, etc.

Neuro Resonas are aspherical lenses with progression on the inner surface, the first to have been developed through the use of neuroscience. The use of these cutting-edge technologies has made it possible to create more ergonomic designs, i.e. able to better adapt to the natural physiology of the body (for example to the movement patterns of the eyes) to facilitate adaptation and improve the wearer's comfort. Thanks to the N-style Wide and Clear design, Neuro Resonas offers a reduction of distortions and aberrations and a better distribution of the astigmatic areas. The field of vision is thus wider and more comfortable compared to conventional progressive lenses. Neuro Resonas can be enhanced with the MYTUNE ENGINE neurotechnology as well.

References:

Tokai Optical exploiting neuroscience in latest progressive design - Insight. (2022). Retrieved 17 October 2023, from https://www.insightnews.com.au/tokai-optical-exploiting-neuroscience-in-latest-progressive-design/

Neuro Progressive - Tokai. (2022). Retrieved 17 October 2023, from https://www.tokai.be/designs/multi-focal/neuro-progressive/

Resonas - Tokai. (2022). Retrieved 17 October 2023, from https://

www.tokai.be/designs/multi-focal/neuro-progressive/resonas/

Feedback from those who purchased neuroscience lenses | Tokai Optical Co., Ltd.. (2022). Retrieved 17 October 2023, from https://www.tokaiopt.com/en/html/advice27/

Ideal comfortable vision selected by the brain. "NEURO SELECT" released on October 1st 2022 | Tokai Optical Co., Ltd.. (2022). Retrieved 17 October 2023, from https://www.tokaiopt.com/en/html/ideal-comfortable-vision-selected-by-the-brain-neuro-select-released-on-october-1st-2022/

Lenskart.com. (n.d.). Lenskart.com - Buy Eyeglasses, Sunglasses and Contact Lens Online. Retrieved October 17, 2023, from https://www.lenskart.com/tokai-lens

TOKAI OPTICAL Co., Ltd. (n.d.). TOKAI OPTICAL Co., Ltd. | A special manufacturer of the latest eyeglass lenses to make the world beautiful. Retrieved October 17, 2023, from https://www.tokaiopt.com/en/

Vision Express. (n.d.). Tokai Lenses – Vision Express. Retrieved October 17, 2023, from https://visionexpress.ph/pages/tokai-lenses

Malaya Optical. (n.d.). Tokai Progressive Lens - Optometrist | Optical Shop. Retrieved October 17, 2023, from https://www.malayaoptical.com/tokai-progressive-lens/

Tokai. (n.d.). Neuro Progressive - Tokai. Retrieved October 17, 2023, from https://www.tokai.be/designs/multi-focal/neuro-progressive/

SEIKO

Seiko Progressive lenses are a type of multifocal lenses that provide clear and comfortable vision for different distances. Seiko offers various progressive lens designs to suit different needs and preferences. Two of the latest products are Neuro Select and Neuro Resonas.

Neuro Select is a new brand of progressive lenses that was launched by Tokai Optical, a subsidiary of Seiko, in October 2022. Neuro Select is based on neuroscience research and aims to provide the ideal comfortable vision selected by the brain. Neuro Select allows users to choose from three situations (daily, town, or home), five grades (super-premium, premium, high, standard, or basic), and three design options (select, I location remix, or my tune engine). Neuro Select also features twin eye modulation technology, which minimizes the difference in image perception between the two eyes and enhances binocular vision. Neuro Select claims to offer comfort that users have never experienced before (Tokai Optical Co., Ltd., 2022).

Neuro Resonas is another new brand of progressive lenses that was launched by Seiko in November 2022. Neuro Resonas is designed to resonate with the user's brain and provide natural and smooth vision. Neuro Resonas uses a new design engine called Easyone WS, which combines double-surface progressive and double-surface aspheric design. Neuro Resonas also incorporates flexible prism thinning, which balances the thickness and prismatic effects of the lenses for better aesthetics and comfort. Neuro Resonas offers four options for users: standard, wide, extra wide, or ultra-wide (Seiko Vision, n.d.).

Both Neuro Select and Neuro Resonas are innovative products that use neuroscience to optimize progressive lens design and performance. They offer customized solutions for users who want to enjoy diverse activities and lifestyles with clear and comfortable vision.

Seiko Progressive lenses are multifocal lenses that provide

clear and comfortable vision at all distances, from near to far. Seiko offers a wide range of progressive lenses, each with different features and benefits to suit different lifestyles and needs. Here are some of the progressive lenses from Seiko's portfolio:

SEIKO Brilliance: A supreme progressive lens that is customized to the wearer's needs and optimized for digital usage. It has a smooth transition between the near, intermediate and far zones, and a wide field of view in each zone. It also reduces distortion and eye fatigue caused by switching between different devices. SEIKO Brilliance is ideal for those who demand precise and luxurious vision at all times.

SEIKO Prime Xceed / Prime X: The high-end progressive lens designs from Seiko that use Twin Eye Modulation Technology (TMT) to enhance binocular vision and balance. TMT minimizes the differences in image perception between the two eyes, which can cause irritation and discomfort in conventional progressive lenses. SEIKO Prime Xceed / Prime X also use Flexible Prism Thinning to balance the thickness and aesthetics of the lenses. SEIKO Prime Xceed is the customized version of SEIKO Prime X, which takes into account the wearer's pupillary distance, vertex distance, pantoscopic tilt, wrap angle, fitting height and frame dimensions. SEIKO Prime Xceed / Prime X are suitable for those who require higher precision, unparalleled quality and bespoke design.

SEIKO Surmount / Surmount Ws: The 100% internal free-form progressive lenses that use complex convex curves on the back surface of the lens to achieve flatter base curves on plus power prescriptions. This reduces the magnification effect and improves the cosmetic appearance of the lenses. SEIKO Surmount / Surmount Ws also have a wide near zone, a smooth progression corridor and a balanced distance zone. They are designed to reduce unwanted astigmatism and distortion in the peripheral areas of the lens. SEIKO Surmount Ws is the newer version of SEIKO Surmount, which has an improved design for wrap frames and sporty activities. SEIKO Surmount / Surmount Ws are recommended for those who want robust and attractive lenses, even with high prescriptions.

SEIKO Sports / Drive / Computer: The specialized progressive lenses that are tailored for specific purposes and environments. SEIKO Sports is designed for outdoor activities and sports, with a wider distance zone, a shorter progression corridor and a dynamic near zone. It also has a high impact resistance and UV protection. SEIKO Drive is designed for driving, with a wider intermediate zone, a longer progression corridor and a reduced near zone. It also has a polarized filter that reduces glare and enhances contrast. SEIKO Computer is designed for computer work, with a wider near zone, a shorter progression corridor and a reduced distance zone. It also has a blue light filter that protects the eyes from digital devices. These lenses are ideal for those who need specific solutions for their hobbies or occupations.

References:

Progressive | Seiko Vision (n.d.). Retrieved October 17, 2023, from https://www.seikovision.com/lenses/progressive/

Which Seiko Progressive Lenses Are Best for Me? (n.d.). Retrieved October 17, 2023, from https://progressive-glasses.com/which-seiko-progressive-lenses-are-best-for-me/

SEIKO Surmount & Surmount Ws - Robertson Optical Laboratories (n.d.). Retrieved October 17, 2023, from http://www.robertsonoptical.com/wp/wp-content/uploads/2016/03/Surmount07601_4pg.pdf

SEIKO progressive lenses at Visio Optical (n.d.). Retrieved October 17, 2023, from https://visiooptical.com/products/lenses/seiko/progressive-lenses/

Seiko Vision. (n.d.). Progressive. Retrieved from https://www.seikovision.com/lenses/progressive/

Tokai Optical Co., Ltd. (2022). Ideal comfortable vision selected by the brain. "NEURO SELECT" was released on October 1st 2022. Retrieved from https://www.tokaiopt.com/en/news/

ideal-comfortable-vision-selected-by-the-brain-neuro-
select-released-on-october-1st-2022/

NIKON

Nikon Progressive lenses are a type of eyeglasses that can correct presbyopia, which is a condition that affects the ability to focus on near objects as people age. Nikon offers a wide range of progressive lenses that can provide superior optical performance, better aesthetics and optimal comfort. Some of the progressive lenses that Nikon offers are:

SeeMax Ultimate: The first progressive lens co-designed with the user based on their unique vision insights for the ultimate viewing experience. It uses a patented algorithm to optimize the lens design according to the user's frame shape, eye parameters, lifestyle and visual preferences. (Nikon Lenswear, n.d.-a)

Presio Master: A progressive lens designed to eliminate visual stress and provide minimal distortions all around. It uses a 3D design technology that takes into account the natural eye movements and the lens position on the face. It also has a wide intermediate zone for smooth transitions between near and far vision. (Nikon Lenswear, n.d.-b)

Presio Power: A dual-power progressive design with a wider intermediate vision for fast adaptation and sharper vision. It uses a dual-power technology that reduces unwanted astigmatism and enhances binocular vision. It also has a balanced near zone for comfortable reading. (Nikon Lenswear, n.d.-c)

Presio W: A dynamic progressive lens with a large viewing area from far to near, pushing the boundaries of vision. It uses a dynamic design technology that adapts to the user's visual behaviour and environment. It also has a wide zone for easy access to digital devices. (Nikon Lenswear, n.d.-d)

References:

Nikon Lenswear. (n.d.-a). SeeMax Ultimate Progressive lenses | Nikon Lenswear. Retrieved December 17, 2021, from https://www.nikonlenswear.com/eyeglasses/progressive-lenses/seemax-ultimate-progressive-lenses/

Nikon Lenswear. (n.d.-b). Presio Master Progressive lenses | Nikon Lenswear. Retrieved December 17, 2021, from https://www.nikonlenswear.com/eyeglasses/progressive-lenses/presio-master-progressive-lenses/

Nikon Lenswear. (n.d.-c). Presio Power Progressive lenses | Nikon Lenswear India. Retrieved December 17, 2021, from https://www.nikonlenswear.com/in/eyeglasses/progressive-lenses/presio-power-progressive-lenses/

Nikon Lenswear. (n.d.-d). Presio W Progressive lenses | Nikon Lenswear India. Retrieved December 17, 2021, from https://www.nikonlenswear.com/in/eyeglasses/progressive-lenses/presio-w-progressive-lenses/

ZEISS

Zeiss by Carl Zeiss Vision is a leading brand of progressive addition lenses (PALs) that offer high-quality vision correction with innovative technologies and features. Some of the Zeiss products are:

Zeiss Individual 2: These lenses are individually designed for each wearer using the wearer's prescription, fitting geometry, frame information, and visual profile. They provide a smooth transition throughout the lens, irrespective of where the wearer is looking. They also incorporate EyeFit and CORE technologies to create a personalized vision experience.

Zeiss Precision Plus: These lenses are suitable for all customers with a near addiction who want sharp vision at any distance. They allow for an unlimited choice of glass frames, and the lens adaptation time is fast. They also incorporate Digital Inside technology that accounts for the typical reading position of digital devices and extends the near zone vertically and horizontally for comfortable reading of any media, whether print or digital.

Zeiss Precision Superb: These lenses are perfectly adapted to the wearer's frame of choice and fitted to their facial anatomy. They also incorporate Digital Inside technology and FrameFit+ technology that ensures the best possible lens fit for any frame shape or size.

Zeiss Precision Pure: These lenses provide fast focus and good dynamic vision all day long. They are suitable for using different media from closer reading distances to further distances. They also incorporate Digital Inside technology and Luminance Design technology that optimises the lens design based on pupil size in different light conditions.

Zeiss DriveSafe: These lenses are designed to meet the vision needs of people who want to feel safer and more comfortable when driving with their everyday lenses. They reduce glare at night, provide better vision in low-light conditions, and enable easy switching of focus between the road, dashboard, rear-view mirror, and side mirrors.

Zeiss Officelens: These lenses are designed to meet the vision needs of people who spend most of their time indoors and require frequent changes of focus at various distances. They provide clear and comfortable vision for near to intermediate distances, up to 4 metres. They also reduce eye strain and neck pain caused by the prolonged use of digital devices.

References:

ZEISS Progressive Individual 2 Lenses. (n.d.). Retrieved October 17, 2023, from https://www.zeiss.com/content/dam/Vision/Vision/en_us/PDF/ECP/ZI2_FitDisp_Guide_051012FNLAppd.pdf

Penczek, M. (2020, December 14). Zeiss Individual 2: An Owner's In-Depth Review. Progressive Glasses. https://progressive-glasses.com/zeiss-individual-2-an-owners-in-depth-review/

ZEISS Progressive lenses. (n.d.). Retrieved October 17, 2023, from https://www.zeiss.co.in/vision-care/eye-care-professionals/lenses/lens-type/progressive-lenses.html

ZEISS Precision Plus Digital Lens. (n.d.). Retrieved October 17, 2023, from https://www.k-optical.com/zeisslens/zeissprecisionplus/zeissprecisionplus.html

ZEISS DriveSafe Lenses. (n.d.). Retrieved October 17, 2023, from https://www.zeiss.com/vision-care/int/better-vision/understanding-vision/drivesafe-lenses.html

ZEISS Office Lenses. (n.d.). Retrieved October 17, 2023, from https://www.zeiss.com/vision-care/int/better-vision/understanding-vision/office-lenses.html

ZEISS

Carl Zeiss Vision (Gradal) progressive lenses are a range of high-quality lenses that offer optimum vision support for the near and far zones. They are tailor-made for the individual needs and preferences of the wearer, ensuring greater comfort, faster adaptation and smooth transitions. The Gradal HS progressive lens, introduced in 1983, was a breakthrough innovation that featured horizontal symmetry (HS) design, which ensured equivalent visual impressions for the right and left eye, as well as comfortable binocular vision (Fürter, 1983). Since then, Carl Zeiss Vision has developed various progressive lens designs based on advanced technologies and research, such as ZEISS SmartLife, ZEISS Precision and ZEISS Intelligence Augmented Design. These lenses are designed to address the visual challenges of modern lifestyles, such as the frequent use of digital devices, dynamic head and eye movements, and different frame choices. They also provide full UV protection and can be made of plastic or glass materials with different refractive indices and thicknesses. Carl Zeiss Vision (Gradal) progressive lenses are suitable for wearers in their 40s and over with a near addition, who want to see details clearly at all distances, without sacrificing style or aesthetics.

References
Fürter, G. (1983). Progressive spectacle lens with horizontal symmetry. U.S. Patent No. 4,402,594. https://patents.google.com/patent/US4402594A/en
ZEISS Progressive lenses. (n.d.). Retrieved October 17, 2023, from https://www.zeiss.co.in/vision-care/spectacle-lenses-from-zeiss/progressive-lenses-portfolio.html
ZEISS Progressive lenses. (n.d.). Retrieved October 17, 2023, from https://www.zeiss.co.uk/vision-care/eye-care-professionals/lenses/lens-type/progressive-lenses.html
How a patent filed by ZEISS set new standards for progressive lenses 30 years ago. (2019, October 16). Retrieved October 17, 2023, from https://www.zeiss.com.au/vision-care/eye-health-and-care/understanding-vision/how-a-patent-filed-by-zeiss-set-new-standards-for-progressive-lenses-30-years-ago.html

ZEISS (Gradal)

Gradal progressive lenses are a type of multifocal lens that correct vision at different distances, from near to far, without any visible lines or segments. They have a gradual change in prescription across the lens, providing a smooth and seamless transition from one power to another. Gradal progressive lenses are suitable for people who have presbyopia, astigmatism, or other refractive errors that affect their ability to see clearly at various ranges.

There are different types of gradal progressive lenses, depending on the design, material, and coating of the lens. Some of the common types are:

Standard progressive lenses: These are the basic and most affordable type of gradal lenses. They have a wide intermediate zone and a narrow reading zone, making them ideal for people who need clear vision for distance and computer use. However, they may cause some distortion or blur in the peripheral areas of the lens.

Computer progressive lenses: These are specially designed for people who spend a lot of time working on digital devices, such as computers, tablets, or smartphones. They have a larger reading zone and a smaller distance zone, allowing for more comfortable and natural eye movements when switching between near and intermediate tasks. They also reduce eye strain and fatigue caused by blue light emitted from screens.

Short corridor progressive lenses: These are made for people who have smaller or narrower frames that cannot accommodate the standard progressive lenses. They have a shorter vertical height and a faster change in prescription, which means they have less distortion and more clarity in the central area of the lens. However, they also have smaller zones for distance, intermediate, and near vision, which may require more head movements to find the optimal focus.

Transition progressive lenses: These are also known as photochromic lenses, as they change their tint according to the amount of light exposure. They are clear indoors and darken outdoors, protecting from UV rays and glare. They are convenient and versatile for people who need vision correction in different lighting conditions.

Premium progressive lenses: These are the most advanced and customized type of gradal lenses. They use digital technology and sophisticated algorithms to create a personalized lens design that matches the individual's eye shape, prescription, frame size, and lifestyle preferences. They offer the widest and clearest fields of vision, with minimal distortion and adaptation time.

Ground-view progressive lenses: These are designed for people who need extra vision support for activities that involve looking down, such as golfing, gardening, or driving. They have an additional power zone at the bottom of the lens that enhances the lower visual field and improves depth perception and contrast sensitivity.

Gradal progressive lenses are available from various brands and manufacturers, such as ZEISS, Essilor, Hoya, Rodenstock, etc. Each brand has its portfolio of products that offer different features and benefits for different needs and preferences. For example:

ZEISS Gradal Individual 2: This is a premium progressive lens that uses ZEISS's patented freeform technology to create a customized lens design based on the wearer's individual eye measurements, frame data, and visual behaviour. It offers high-definition vision in all directions and distances, with up to 50% larger fields of view than conventional progressive lenses.

Essilor Varilux X Series: This is a premium progressive lens that uses Essilor's Xtend technology to extend the wearer's near vision range by up to 50 cm. It allows the wearer to see multiple objects clearly at arm's length without having to move their head or eyes excessively. It also reduces image distortions and enhances contrast and colour perception.

Hoya Lifestyle 3: This is a premium progressive lens that uses Hoya's Binocular Harmonization Technology to balance the prescription between both eyes and optimize the binocular visual performance. It also uses Hoya's Integrated Double Surface Design to reduce aberrations and increase visual acuity in all zones of the lens.

Rodenstock Impression FreeSign 3: This is a premium progressive lens that uses Rodenstock's Eye Lens Technology to create a tailor-made lens design based on the wearer's biometric data, such as eye length, corneal shape, pupil size, etc. It also uses Rodenstock's FreeSign technology to allow the wearer to choose their preferred near vision zone from three options: balanced, dynamic, or intensive.

References:
Vision Center (2023). Progressive Lenses (Types, Pros & Cons). Retrieved from https://www.visioncenter.org/eyeglasses/progressive-lenses/
Healthline (2023). What Are Progressive Lenses: Types & Benefits. Retrieved from https://www.healthline.com/health/what-are-progressive-lenses
All About Vision (2019). Progressive Lenses: No-line Multifocals for a Younger You. Retrieved from https://www.allaboutvision.com/lenses/progressives.htm
Specsavers (n.d.). What are progressive lenses? Retrieved from https://www.specsavers.co.uk/help-and-faqs/what-are-progressive-lenses
ZEISS (n.d.). ZEISS Gradal Individual 2. Retrieved from https://www.zeiss.com/vision-care/int/eye-care-professionals/products/spectacle-lenses/progressive-lenses/gradal-individual-2.html
Essilor (n.d.). Varilux X Series. Retrieved from https://www.essilor.co.uk/varilux/varilux-x-series
Hoya (n.d.). Lifestyle 3. Retrieved

from https://www.hoyavision.com/discover-products/
for-eye-care-professionals/corrective-lenses/progressive-
lenses/lifestyle-3/

Rodenstock (n.d.). Impression FreeSign 3. Retrieved
from https://www.rodenstock.com/com/en/progressive-
lenses/impression-freesign-3.html

Deutsche Augenoptik AG (DAO)

Deutsche Augenoptik AG (DAO) is a leading supplier of high-quality and individual lenses, including progressive lenses. Progressive lenses allow for optimal vision at different distances, without disturbing transitions or edges. DAO offers various progressive lenses that are tailored to the needs and requirements of customers. DAO's progressive lenses include:

UP by DAO: A price-attractive line of glasses that offers high quality and a modern design. UP by DAO is available in various materials, colours and coatings and is suitable for all common versions.

PERFORMER: A sports brand designed specifically for active people. PERFORMER offers dynamic vision, high tolerance and reliable protection against UV rays, blue light and scratches. PERFORMER can be used in various sports, such as golf, cycling or skiing.

Noflex: A hyperreflection that reduces the reflections on the glasses and ensures a clear and contrasting vision. noflex is especially suitable for people who work a lot at the screen or drive at night. noflex is compatible with all DAO progressive lenses.

UV420: A blue light filter that protects the eyes from harmful blue-violet light emanating from digital devices or artificial light sources. UV420 improves eye comfort and well-being and can reduce the risk of eye fatigue, headache or sleep disorders. UV420 is compatible with all DAO progressive lenses.

References:
Startseite - DAO - Deutsche Augenoptik AG. (n.d.). Retrieved October 17, 2023, from https://www.dao-ag.de/
Progressive Glasses Brands. (n.d.). Retrieved October 17, 2023, from https://progressive-glasses.com/progressive-glasses-brands/
ZEISS Progressive lenses. (n.d.). Retrieved October 17, 2023, from https://www.zeiss.co.in/vision-care/eye-care-professionals/lenses/lens-type/progressive-lenses.html

Frame Tec

Frame Tec progressive lenses are a range of advanced digital progressive lenses that offer an outstanding visual experience for customers who need correction for near and distance vision. Frame Tec progressive lenses are powered by camber-finished lenses, which provide spacious reading zones, improved peripheral vision, an expanded Rx range, better-looking lenses in many materials, and patient-preferred near vision performance (Lens Options - Lenstec Optical Group, n.d.). Frame Tec progressive lenses are also perfectly adapted to the wearer's frame of choice and facial anatomy, using ZEISS SmartView 2.0 technology and ZEISS Intelligence Augmented Design technology based on applied research of today's lifestyle, visual behaviour, and age-related visual needs (ZEISS Progressive lenses, n.d.). Frame Tec progressive lenses are suitable for customers who want to see details clearly at all distances, without sacrificing comfort, and who use different media from closer reading distances to further distances. Frame Tec progressive lenses also eliminate the visible line in the middle of the lens, which hides the fact that the user needs reading glasses (Progressive Lenses for Clear Vision at All Distance | Essilor India, n.d.). Frame Tec progressive lenses are available in plastic and glass materials, with various additions and coatings to suit different needs and preferences.

References

Lens Options - Lenstec Optical Group. (n.d.). Retrieved October 17, 2023, from http://lenstecopticalgroup.co.uk/lens-options/

Progressive Lenses for Clear Vision at All Distance | Essilor India. (n.d.). Retrieved October 17, 2023, from https://www.essilorindia.com/products/progressive-lenses

ZEISS Progressive lenses. (n.d.). Retrieved October 17, 2023, from https://www.zeiss.co.in/vision-care/eye-care-professionals/lenses/lens-type/progressive-lenses.html

Eugen Stratemyer GmbH & Co.KG

Eugen Stratemyer GmbH & Co.KG is a German company that produces high-quality progressive lenses for various applications. Progressive lenses are lenses that have a smooth transition from distance to near vision, without any visible lines or segments. Progressive lenses can provide a natural and comfortable vision for people who need correction for both distance and near vision, such as presbyopes.

According to their website, Eugen Stratemyer GmbH & Co.KG offers a wide range of progressive lenses, including:

EYEfinity: The new progressive lens line with image stabilization, which reduces the effects of head movements and provides a stable and clear vision in all directions.

EverClean: The new cleaning layer with a water-repellent effect, which makes the lenses easy to clean and resistant to dirt, dust, and fingerprints.

BEST Nature: The new subtle reflection colour, reduces glare and enhances contrast and colour perception.

Balance-Filter: A special filter that reduces the impact of blue light and provides relaxation for light-sensitive eyes.

STAR-OPTIMAL Innovation: A comprehensive solution for cataract surgery patients, which includes progressive lenses, sunglasses, and reading glasses.

Eugen Stratemyer GmbH & Co.KG also provides progressive lenses for digital devices, driving, sports, and occupational safety. Their progressive lenses are made in Germany, with high-quality materials and advanced technology. They are exclusively available through traditional opticians.

References:

Stratemeyer: Startseite. (n.d.). Retrieved October 17, 2023, from https://www.stratemeyer.eu/

Progressive Glasses Brands. (n.d.). Retrieved October 17, 2023, from https://progressive-glasses.com/progressive-glasses-brands/

Eugen Stratemeyer GmbH & Co. KG Company Profile | Bochum, Nordrhein-Westfalen, Germany | Competitors, Financials & Contacts - Dun & Bradstreet. (n.d.). Retrieved October 17, 2023, from https://www.dnb.com/business-directory/company-profiles.eugen_stratemeyer_gmbh__co_kg.c8a7ff6388206 19a74d1e30421c3c77.html

Kodak

Kodak progressive lenses are available in different designs and materials to suit your lifestyle and vision needs. Some of the Kodak progressive lenses are

Kodak Unique II HD Lens: This lens is designed to provide

high-definition vision with minimal distortion and adaptation issues. It uses a digital back surface that takes into account the front progressive design, the frame shape, the fitting measurements and the prescription. It also offers a wide range of corridor lengths and fitting heights to fit various frames.

Kodak Easy Lens: This lens is designed to provide easy adaptation and comfortable vision for first-time progressive lens wearers. It has a soft design that reduces peripheral blur and swim effect. It also has a balanced near zone that provides a clear reading vision.

Kodak Precise Lens: This lens is designed to provide precise vision with enhanced contrast and clarity. It uses a patented progressive design that optimizes the optical performance of each lens power. It also has a short corridor option for smaller frames.

Kodak SoftWear Lens: This lens is designed to provide comfortable computer viewing and relief from eye strain. It has a digital design that reduces distortion and provides a wider intermediate zone. It also has a soft near zone that allows for easy transition from computer to near tasks.

References:
Kodak Lens India. (n.d.). Retrieved October 17, 2023, from https://www.kodaklens.in/
Kodak Progressive Lenses - Correcting for Vision at Any Distance. (n.d.). Retrieved October 17, 2023, from https://www.kodaklens.us/products/kodak-progressive-lenses/
Kodak Progressive Lenses – A Buyer's Guide. (2020, December 14). Retrieved October 17, 2023, from https://progressive-glasses.com/kodak-progressive-lenses-a-buyers-guide/
KODAK PROGRESSIVE LENS DISPENSING AID. (n.d.). Retrieved October 17, 2023, from https://www.kodaklens.us/wp-content/uploads/2017/04/KODAK-Precise-Digital-Lens-Dispensing-Guide.pdf

Leica

Leica Eyecare offers a range of premium progressive lenses that correct presbyopia and provide sharp vision at all distances. The VARIOVID® progressive lenses are designed with the latest calculation and production methods to optimize visual ranges based on individual visual acuity and visual habits. They also have a high spontaneous tolerance, meaning that the eyes can quickly adapt to the new vision. The VARIOVID® progressive lenses are available in different categories, each with a particular feature, such as large usable areas, stable visual acuity, natural vision, or reduced unwanted astigmatism. The VARIOVID® progressive lenses also come with options for different activities, such as driving, sports, or photography. The VARIOVID® progressive lenses are made of AQUADURA® VISION, a coating that protects the lenses from scratches, dust, water, and reflections.

References:

Premium VARIOVID® progressive lenses | LEICA EYECARE. (n.d.). Retrieved October 17, 2023, from https://leica-eyecare.com/en/spectacle-lenses/the-progressive-lens/

Ophthalmic Lenses | Leica Camera AG. (n.d.). Retrieved October 17, 2023, from https://leica-camera.com/en-int/ophthalmic-lenses

Ophthalmic Lenses | Leica Camera US. (n.d.). Retrieved October 17, 2023, from https://leica-camera.com/en-US/ophthalmic-lenses

Luxexcel

Luxexcel is a company that specializes in 3D printing prescription lenses for smart glasses. Luxexcel's VisionPlatform 7 is a technology that enables the integration of various objects, such as waveguides, holographic optical elements, and liquid crystal foils, into the 3D printing process of lenses. This allows for the creation of thin, lightweight, and customizable lenses that can project images from electronics to the eye. Luxexcel's VisionPlatform 7 can print lenses with different powers, diameters, and designs, such as single-vision lenses and multifocal progressive lenses. Luxexcel's VisionPlatform 7 also prints critical features, such as the air gap required for a waveguide, and a hard coating to protect the integrated technologies.

References:

Heimgartner, J. (2021, August 10). Luxexcel's VisionPlatform 7 Makes Prescription Smart Glasses a Reality. Engineering.com. https://www.engineering.com/story/luxexcels-visionplatform-7-makes-prescription-smart-glasses-a-reality

Manufactur3D. (2021, July 18). Luxexcel launches VisionPlatform™ 7 for Manufacturing of Prescription Smart Lenses. Manufactur3D. https://manufactur3dmag.com/luxexcel-launches-visionplatform-7-for-manufacturing-of-prescription-smart-lenses/

Auganix. (2021, July 15). Luxexcel launches platform for manufacturing of prescription lenses for AR smart glasses. Auganix. https://www.auganix.org/luxexcel-launches-platform-for-manufacturing-of-prescription-lenses-for-ar-smart-glasses/

Scott, S. (2020, August 29). Luxexcel advances 3D printing technology for ophthalmic lenses. 3D Printing Industry.

https://3dprintingindustry.com/news/luxexcel-advances-3d-printing-technology-for-ophthalmic-lenses-149435/

Molitch-Hou, M. (2021, July 27). Luxexcel Announces Platform for 3D Printing Prescription Lenses for Smartglasses. 3DPrint.com. https://3dprint.com/283560/luxexcel-announces-visionplatform-7-for-3d-printing-prescription-smartglass-lenses/

Nordhorn Optic

Nordhorn Optic is a German manufacturer of progressive lenses that offers a range of products for different visual needs and preferences. According to Progressive Glasses, Nordhorn Optic is one of the many brands that produce progressive lenses, which are lenses that have no lines separating the different lens strengths, yet they provide the user with clear vision at all distances (Progressive Glasses, 2020). Some of the benefits of progressive lenses are:

- They allow both head and eyes to stay in a natural and comfortable position when looking at objects in the distance, the intermediate zone and close up.
- They eliminate the visible line in the middle of the lens, which can be aesthetically unappealing and reveal the need for reading glasses.
- They have a smooth and seamless progression of lens power that runs vertically down each lens, providing a more natural depth focus than bifocals.

Nordhorn Optic's progressive lenses are available in different materials, such as plastic, polycarbonate, trivex and high-index. They also have different designs, such as balanced, dynamic, harmonious and individual, which cater to different lifestyles and visual demands. For example, the balanced design is suitable for users who need a balanced vision for near and far distances, while the dynamic design is ideal for users who are active and need a wider field of view for dynamic activities. The harmony design is optimized for users who spend a lot of time on digital devices and need a comfortable vision for intermediate and near distances. The individual design is customized for each user's specific prescription, frame and eye measurements, providing the best possible vision quality and comfort.

Nordhorn Optic's progressive lenses can be combined with various coatings and filters to enhance their performance and protection. For instance, they can have anti-reflective coating to reduce glare and reflections, scratch-resistant coating to prevent damage, UV protection to block harmful rays, blue light filter to reduce eye strain from digital screens, photochromic coating to adjust to different light conditions, polarized coating to eliminate horizontal glare from surfaces like water or snow, etc.

To summarize, Nordhorn Optic is a brand of progressive lenses that offers a variety of products for different visual needs and preferences. Progressive lenses are lenses that have no lines separating the different lens strengths, yet they provide the user with clear vision at all distances. They have several benefits over bifocals or multiple pairs of glasses, such as natural and comfortable head and eye posture, aesthetic appeal, smooth and seamless transition of lens power and more natural depth focus. Nordhorn Optic's progressive lenses are available in different materials, designs, coatings and filters to suit each user's requirements.

References

Progressive Glasses. (2020). Progressive Glasses Brands. Retrieved from https://progressive-glasses.com/progressive-glasses-brands/

Optovision

Optovision Progressive Lenses are a type of glasses that provide clear vision at any distance, from near to far, without any visible lines separating the different lens strengths. They are designed to fit the individual eyes and viewing habits of the wearer and offer comfortable, wide fields of vision in all situations. Optovision Progressive Lenses are manufactured in Germany using free-form technology, which ensures high precision and quality. Optovision Progressive Lenses can also be customized for specific purposes, such as driving, sports, or indoor work.

According to the optoVision website, Optovision Progressive Lenses have the following features:
- Continuous and seamless transitions between looking at a tablet with razor-sharp vision and a relaxing gaze at the horizon
- Immediate sharp vision and natural head and body posture
- Prevention of headaches or muscular tension at work
- Extra protection by up to 11 layers of strong i-Protection ® + coatings
- Prescription sunglasses with self-tinting sun protection

Optovision Progressive Lenses are one of the many options available for people who need glasses for different distances. They are suitable for those who value convenience, comfort, and quality in their vision correction. However, they may not be the best choice for everyone, as some people may experience adaptation difficulties, distortion, or reduced peripheral vision with progressive lenses. Therefore, it is important to consult with an ophthalmic optician before deciding on the type of glasses that best suit one's needs and preferences.

References
optoVision. (n.d.). Progressive lenses. Retrieved October 17, 2023, from https://www.optovision.com/en/lenses/lens-types/progressive-lenses.html
optoVision. (n.d.). Lens types. Retrieved October 17, 2023, from

https://www.optovision.com/en/lenses/lens-types.html
Vision Center. (2023, October 13). Progressive lenses (types, pros, cons & costs). Retrieved October 17, 2023, from https://www.visioncenter.org/eyeglasses/progressive-lenses/
Essilor India. (n.d.). Progressive lenses for clear vision at all distance. Retrieved October 17, 2023, from https://www.essilorindia.com/products/progressive-lenses

Rupp + Hubrach (R+H)

Rupp + Hubrach (R+H) is a German company that produces high-quality ophthalmic lenses for various needs and preferences. One of their products is the progressive lens, which offers a smooth transition from near to far vision without visible lines or distortions. Progressive lenses are suitable for people who need correction for both presbyopia and myopia, hyperopia, or astigmatism.

R+H offers different types of progressive lenses, such as:

SiiA: A personalized progressive lens that adapts to the individual eye parameters, frame shape, and wearing position of the wearer. SiiA provides a wide field of vision, natural posture, and high visual comfort in all situations (Rupp & Hubrach Brillenglas, n.d.-a).

Selectal: A standard progressive lens that is easy to fit and wear. Selectal has a balanced design that ensures good vision at all distances and reduces unwanted astigmatism (Rupp & Hubrach Brillenglas, n.d.-b).

Sports: A progressive lens that is specially designed for sports activities. Sports has a large distance zone, a dynamic intermediate zone, and a small near zone. It also has a high impact resistance and can be combined with various tints and coatings for optimal performance (Optician Online, 2006).

R+H progressive lenses are coated with a multilayered antireflective coating that reduces glare, enhances contrast, and improves visual acuity. The coating also has a low light reflection factor in both photopic and scotopic vision, which means it works well in bright and dark conditions (Rupp + Hubrach Optik GmbH, 2018). Moreover, R+H progressive lenses can be customized with PURLUX, an anti-reflective coating that has no residual colour and provides a pure and clear appearance (Envision, n.d.).

R+H progressive lenses are a reliable and innovative choice for people who want to enjoy clear and comfortable vision at all distances and in all situations.

References

Envision. (n.d.). PURLUX: Pure luxury for lenses. https://envisionmagazine.ca/purlux-pure-luxury-for-lenses/

Optician Online. (2006, August 30). Rupp + Hubrach offers Sports lens. https://www.opticianonline.net/content/news/rupp-plus-hubrach-offers-sports-lens

Rupp & Hubrach Brillenglas. (n.d.-a). SiiA - Rupp and Hubrach - Eyelenses. https://www.rh-brillenglas.de/en/seeing-through-new-eyes/world-of-vision/progressive-lenses/siia

Rupp & Hubrach Brillenglas. (n.d.-b). Selectal - Rupp and Hubrach - Eyelenses. https://www.rh-brillenglas.de/en/seeing-through-new-eyes/world-of-vision/progressive-lenses/selectal

Rupp + Hubrach Optik GmbH. (2018). U.S. Patent No. 10,072,789. U.S. Patent and Trademark Office.

Vision Ease

Vision Ease is a global ophthalmic lens manufacturer that offers a range of progressive lenses for different needs and preferences. Progressive lenses are a type of multifocal lens that provides a smooth transition from distance to near vision without visible lines or segments. They can correct near-sightedness, farsightedness, and astigmatism, as well as presbyopia, which is the age-related loss of ability to focus on close objects (Healthline, 2018). Some of the progressive lenses available from Vision Ease are:

Novel 1.50 Progressive: This is an all-purpose conventional progressive lens with a 16.5 mm minimum fitting height and a 13 mm corridor. It has a wearer-validated, balanced design that provides vision as good as or better than backside digital lenses across 80% of the Rx range. It also has a corridor inset that varies by base curve and optimal viewing area placement for natural head and eye movement (VisionEase, n.d.-a).

Coppertone Polarized Lenses in Trivex material: This is a new offering that combines the leading sun protection of Coppertone with durable, lightweight Trivex material. It blocks 100% of UVA and UVB rays, as well as harmful blue light. It also enhances colour perception, contrast, and visual comfort in bright light conditions. It is available in grey and brown colours and single-vision and progressive designs (VisionEase, 2018).

Photochromic Brown: This is a photochromic lens that adapts to changing light conditions by darkening outdoors and clearing indoors. It has a brown colour that enhances contrast and depth perception, as well as reduces glare and eye fatigue. It is compatible with most frames and coatings and has a fast activation and fade-back time. It is also available in grey colour and single-vision and progressive designs (VisionEase, 2017).

References
Healthline. (2018, November 30). What are progressive lenses: Types, benefits, and more. https://www.healthline.com/health/what-are-progressive-lenses

VisionEase. (n.d.-a). VISION EASE Novel 1.50 Progressive -

VisionEase. https://visionease.com/products/vision-ease-novel-1-50-progressive/

VisionEase. (n.d.-b). VISION EASE | A Global Ophthalmic Lens Manufacturer. https://visionease.com/

VisionEase. (2017, September 13). VISION EASE Broadens its High-Performance Photochromic Line with New Brown Lenses [Press release]. https://visionease.com/vision-ease-broadens-high-performance-photochromic-line-new-brown-lenses/

VisionEase. (2018, March 15). VISION EASE introduces Coppertone® Polarized Lenses in Trivex® material [Press release]. https://visionease.com/vision-ease-introduces-coppertone-polarized-lenses-trivex-material/

GLOBAL PROGRESSIVE LENS USAGE PATTERN

Progressive lenses are widely used by people who have presbyopia, a condition that affects the ability to focus on close objects as one age. According to a report by Grand View Research, the global progressive lenses market size was valued at USD 18.3 billion in 2019 and is expected to grow at a compound annual growth rate (CAGR) of 4.2% from 2020 to 2027. The report also states that the major factors driving the demand for progressive lenses are the increasing prevalence of presbyopia, the rising awareness about eye health, the growing preference for aesthetic and comfortable eyewear, and the technological advancements in lens design and manufacturing.

One of the leading brands in the progressive lens industry is Essilor, a French company that offers a wide range of products for different needs and lifestyles. Essilor's progressive lenses portfolio includes:

Varilux: The first progressive lens brand, launched in 1959, that provides sharp and natural vision at any distance and in any situation. Varilux lenses are customized to each wearer's prescription, eye shape, frame, and behaviour using advanced technologies such as W.A.V.E. Technology 2, Nanoptix, Synchroneyes, and EyeCode.

Eyezen: A progressive lens brand designed for digital device users, who spend an average of seven hours a day looking at screens. Eyezen lenses help reduce eye strain and fatigue by providing enhanced contrast and clarity for near vision, as well as protection from blue light emitted by digital devices.

Transitions: A progressive lens brand that adapts to changing light conditions, from clear indoors to dark outdoors. Transition lenses block 100% of UV rays and help filter harmful blue light from both natural and artificial sources. Transitions lenses are available in different colours and styles to suit different preferences and personalities.

Crizal: A progressive lens brand that offers superior protection from glare, scratches, smudges, dust, water, and UV rays. Crizal lenses also enhance the aesthetics and durability of eyeglasses by providing a clear and transparent coating that is easy to clean and maintain.

Conclusion

Progressive lenses are a type of multifocal lenses that provide a smooth transition from near to far vision correction. They are designed to mimic the natural function of the eye and to reduce the need for switching between different pairs of glasses. Progressive lenses are widely used by people who have presbyopia, a condition that affects the ability to focus on close objects as one age. The global progressive lenses market size is expected to grow at a CAGR of 4.2% from 2020 to 2027, driven by the increasing prevalence of presbyopia, the rising awareness about eye health, the growing preference for aesthetic and comfortable eyewear, and the technological advancements in lens design and manufacturing. Essilor is one of the leading brands in the progressive lens industry, offering a wide range of products for different needs and lifestyles, such as Varilux, Eyezen, Transitions, and Crizal.

References
Essilor. (n.d.-a). Varilux progressive lenses. Retrieved October 17, 2023, from https://www.essilor.com/en/brands/varilux/

Essilor. (n.d.-b). Eyezen glasses for digital device users. Retrieved October 17, 2023, from https://www.essilor.com/en/brands/eyezen/

Essilor. (n.d.-c). Transitions adaptive lenses. Retrieved October 17, 2023, from https://www.essilor.com/en/brands/transitions/

Essilor. (n.d.-d). Crizal anti-reflective lenses. Retrieved October 17, 2023, from https://www.essilor.com/en/brands/crizal/

Grand View Research. (2020). Progressive Lenses Market Size, Share & Trends Analysis Report By Design (Standard Progressive Lenses, Short Corridor Progressive Lenses), By Distribution Channel (Online, Offline), By Region, And Segment Forecasts, 2020 - 2027. Retrieved October 17, 2023, from https://www.grandviewresearch.com/industry-analysis/progressive-lenses-market

Holden, B. A., Fricke, T. R., Wilson, D. A., Jong, M., Naidoo, K. S., Sankaridurg, P., ... & Resnikoff, S. (2016). Global prevalence of myopia and high myopia and temporal trends from 2000 through 2050. Ophthalmology, 123(5), 1036-1042.

GLOBAL VS. INDIAN PAL USAGE PATTERN

According to a market report by Arizton, the global progressive lenses market size was valued at USD 29.90 billion in 2021 and is expected to reach USD 38.64 billion by 2027, growing at a CAGR of 4.37% during the forecast period. Progressive lenses are multifocal lenses that allow smooth, clear vision from near to far with one lens, without image jumps or transitions. They are a unique feat of optical technology that requires a lot of know-how, optical calculation and exact knowledge of the wearer's parameters. Progressive lenses are suitable for people who need corrective lenses to see distant and close objects, such as those with refractive errors like myopia, hyperopia, astigmatism and presbyopia.

One of the leading brands in progressive lenses is ZEISS, which offers four types of progressive lens designs: Individual 2, Superb, Plus and Pure. These designs take into account the wearer's parameters, such as visual habits and anatomical data, to provide outstanding visual comfort and quick adaptation. ZEISS progressive lenses also feature innovative technologies, such as Digital Inside Technology, which optimizes near vision for digital devices; Precision Technology, which ensures high-definition vision in all light conditions; and UVProtect Technology, which protects the eyes from harmful UV rays up to 400 nm.

PROGRESSIVE LENSES: A COMPARISON

*Progressive Lenses: A Comparison
of ZEISS Products*

Progressive lenses are a popular choice for people who need corrective lenses to see distant and close objects, such as those with refractive errors like myopia, hyperopia, astigmatism and presbyopia (Arizton, 2022). Progressive lenses are a unique feat of optical technology that require a lot of know-how, optical calculation and exact knowledge of the wearer's parameters (ZEISS, n.d.-a). ZEISS is one of the leading brands in progressive lenses, offering four types of progressive lens designs: Individual 2, Superb, Plus and Pure (ZEISS, n.d.-b). These designs differ in the level of customization and personalization they offer to the wearer. This chapter will compare the features and benefits of each design and provide recommendations for choosing the best progressive lens for different needs and preferences.

Individual 2

Individual 2 is the most customized progressive lens design from ZEISS. It takes into account the wearer's prescription, frame choice, face shape, eye movement and visual behaviour to create a tailor-made lens that provides optimal vision in all distances and directions (ZEISS, n.d.-c). Individual 2 also features Digital Inside Technology, which optimizes near vision for digital devices; Precision Technology, which ensures high-definition vision in all light conditions; and UVProtect Technology, which protects the eyes from harmful UV rays up to 400 nm (ZEISS, n.d.-c). Individual 2 is recommended for people who want the highest level of personalization and comfort in their progressive lenses.

Superb

Superb is a high-performance progressive lens design from ZEISS that provides excellent vision quality and adaptation. It takes into account the wearer's prescription, frame choice and eye movement to create a balanced lens that provides clear vision in all distances and directions (ZEISS, n.d.-d). Superb also features Digital Inside Technology, Precision Technology and UVProtect Technology (ZEISS, n.d.-d). Superb is recommended for people who want a reliable and versatile progressive lens that adapts to their lifestyle.

Plus

Plus is a standard progressive lens design from ZEISS that provides good vision quality and adaptation. It takes into account the wearer's prescription and frame choice to create a comfortable lens that provides clear vision at all distances (ZEISS, n.d.-e). Plus also features Digital Inside Technology and UVProtect Technology (ZEISS, n.d.-e). Plus is recommended for people who want a simple and affordable progressive lens that meets their basic needs.

Pure

Pure is a basic progressive lens design from ZEISS that provides satisfactory vision quality and adaptation. It takes into account the wearer's prescription to create an easy-to-use lens that provides clear vision at all distances (ZEISS,n.d.-f). Pure also features UVProtect Technology (ZEISS,n.d.-f). Pure is recommended for people who want a low-cost progressive lens that offers decent performance.

Conclusion

Progressive lenses are a type of multifocal lens that provides smooth, clear vision from near to far with one lens. ZEISS offers four types of progressive lens designs: Individual 2, Superb, Plus and Pure. These designs differ in the level of customization and personalization they offer to the wearer, as well as the technologies they feature. Depending on the wearer's needs and preferences, they can choose the best progressive lens for them from ZEISS's range of products.

References

Arizton. (2022). Progressive lenses market - global outlook & forecast 2022-2027. https://www.arizton.com/market-reports/progressive-lenses-market

ZEISS. (n.d.-a). All about varifocals. https://www.zeiss.co.in/vision-care/better-vision/help-me-choose/all-about-varifocals.html

ZEISS. (n.d.-b). How do I find the right progressive lenses? https://www.zeiss.co.in/vision-care/better-vision/understanding-vision/how-do-i-find-the-right-progressive-lenses-.html

ZEISS. (n.d.-c). ZEISS progressive individual 2. https://www.zeiss.co.in/vision-care/better-vision/understanding-vision/zeiss-progressive-individual-2.html

ZEISS. (n.d.-d). ZEISS progressive superb. https://www.zeiss.co.in/vision-care/better-vision/understanding-vision/zeiss-progressive-superb.html

ZEISS. (n.d.-e). ZEISS progressive plus. https://www.zeiss.co.in/vision-care/better-vision/understanding-vision/zeiss-progressive-plus.html

ZEISS. (n.d.-f). ZEISS progressive pure. https://www.zeiss.co.in/vision-care/better-vision/understanding-vision/zeiss-progressive-pure.html

FRAME SELECTION TECHNICAL CRITERIA

The width of the frame: The frame should not be wider than the face, as this can cause unwanted reflections and glare on the back surface of the lenses. The frame should also match the pupillary distance of the wearer so that the optical centres of the lenses align with the eyes.

The height of the frame: The frame should have enough vertical space to accommodate the different zones of the progressive lenses. The distance zone should be at least 10 mm above the pupil, and the near zone should be at least 18 mm below the pupil. The frame should also have a minimum height of 28 mm to ensure adequate cut-out.

The angles of the frame: The frame should have a moderate pantoscopic tilt (about 8 degrees) and a slight wrap angle (about 6 degrees) to follow the natural curvature of the face. These angles help to reduce distortion and aberration in the peripheral vision and to optimize the position of the corridor and reading area.

The weight of the frame: The frame should be lightweight and comfortable, as progressive lenses tend to be heavier than single-vision lenses. The frame should also have a good balance and fit, to avoid slipping or sliding on the nose.

In addition to these factors, the frame selection for progressive lenses should also take into account the prescription, lifestyle, and preferences of the wearer. Different types of progressive lenses have different designs and features, such as wider or narrower corridors, shorter or longer progression lengths, and customized or standardized parameters. Some progressive lenses are more suitable for certain activities, such as reading, driving, or working on a computer. Some progressive lenses are also more compatible with certain frames, such as rimless, semi-rimless, or full-rim frames.

One example of a progressive lens that offers a wide range of options and flexibility is the Varilux X Series from Essilor. This lens is designed to provide sharp and dynamic vision in any situation, especially at near and intermediate distances. It uses Xtend technology to extend the depth of field and reduce head movements. It also uses Nanoptix technology to reduce distortion and sway sensations. It also uses Synchroneyes technology to enhance binocular vision and widen the visual fields. Varilux X Series can be customized according to the wearer's prescription, measurements, frame, and behaviour.

The reference list is as follows:

Clearly. (n.d.). What are the best frames for progressive lenses? Retrieved October 17, 2023, from https://www.clearly.ca/thelook/the-best-frames-for-progressive-lenses

Essilor. (n.d.). Varilux X Series. Retrieved October 17, 2023, from https://www.essilor.com/en/progressive-lenses/varilux/varilux-x-series/

Opticampus. (n.d.). Progressive lens dispensing. Retrieved October 17, 2023, from http://opticampus.opti.vision/files/progressive_lens_dispensing.pdf

AI-DESIGNED PROGRESSIVE LENSES : A NEW PARADIGM IN VISION CORRECTION

Progressive lenses are a type of multifocal lens that provide a smooth transition from distance to near vision, without the visible lines or segments of traditional bifocals or trifocals. Progressive lenses are widely used by presbyopes, people who have difficulty focusing on close objects due to age-related changes in the eye. However, not all progressive lenses are created equal. The design and quality of progressive lenses can affect the visual performance, comfort and satisfaction of the wearer.

In recent years, a new generation of progressive lenses has emerged, based on artificial intelligence (AI) technology. AI-designed progressive lenses use advanced algorithms and data analysis to optimize the lens design for each wearer, taking into account their prescription, eye measurements, frame parameters, lifestyle preferences and visual needs. AI-designed progressive lenses aim to provide a more personalized and customized vision correction solution, compared to conventional progressive lenses that are based on standard or average parameters.

Technical Design

The technical design of AI-designed progressive lenses involves several steps. First, the wearer's prescription and eye measurements are obtained using a digital device that captures the eye's shape, size, position and movements. Second, the wearer's frame parameters are measured using a 3D scanner that records the frame's shape, size and position on the face. Third, the wearer's lifestyle preferences and visual needs are assessed using a questionnaire that covers various aspects such as reading habits, computer use, driving frequency, sports activities and hobbies. Fourth, based on these inputs, an AI algorithm generates a unique lens design for each eye, optimizing the lens power distribution, surface curvature, thickness and weight. Fifth, the lens design is transferred to a computer-aided manufacturing system that produces the lens using high-precision tools and materials.

How Does It Work?

AI-designed progressive lenses work by providing a smooth and continuous change in lens power from distance to near vision, without any abrupt jumps or distortions. The lens power is adjusted according to the wearer's eye movements and gaze direction, ensuring clear and comfortable vision at all distances and directions. AI-designed progressive lenses also reduce or eliminate some of the common problems associated with conventional progressive lenses, such as peripheral blur, image swim, adaptation difficulties and reduced fields of view. AI-designed progressive lenses achieve this by minimizing unwanted astigmatism and prismatic effects that occur when the eye moves away from the optical centre of the lens. AI-designed progressive lenses also take into account the wearer's frame parameters and facial anatomy, ensuring a better fit and alignment of the lens on the eye.

Market Availability India
& Global Market

AI-designed progressive lenses are currently available in

India and in several other countries around the world. Some of the leading brands that offer AI-designed progressive lenses are Essilor (Varilux X series), Zeiss (Zeiss Individual 2), Hoya (Hoyalux iD MyStyle V+), Rodenstock (Impression FreeSign 3) and Shamir (Shamir Autograph Intelligence). These brands differ in their specific algorithms, data sources, manufacturing processes and product features, but they all share the common goal of providing a more personalized and customized vision correction solution for presbyopes.

SOME SIGNIFICANT AI-DESIGNED PROGRESSIVE ADDITION LENSES

Essilor: Varilux X series

The Varilux X series is Essilor's latest generation of AI-designed progressive lenses, launched in 2017. The Varilux X series uses Essilor's patented Xtend technology, which extends the wearer's near vision zone by up to 50%, compared to conventional progressive lenses. The Varilux X series also uses Essilor's Nanoptix technology, which reduces image swim by up to 90%, compared to conventional progressive lenses. The Varilux X series is available in four designs: Varilux Xclusive 4D (the most personalized design), Varilux Xtrack (optimized for digital devices), Varilux Xfit (optimized for sports) and Varilux Xdesign (optimized for fashion).

Varilux XR

Varilux XR Series from Essilor, which is the first eye-responsive progressive lens powered by behavioural AI. The lens design goes beyond prescription and eye physiology to consider the wearer's visual behaviour, which is predicted by a behavioural modelling system that analyzes over 1 million data points from exclusive research, wearer tests in real life, and wearer behavioural and postural measurements in-store. The lens also features XR-motion technology, which optimizes binocular vision and precise positioning of the focus zones, providing instant sharpness even in motion. The lens is engineered with environmental consciousness in mind, from its engineering to its packaging (EssilorLuxottica, 2023).

Zeiss: Zeiss Individual 2

The Zeiss Individual 2 is Zeiss's flagship product of AI-designed progressive lenses, launched in 2012. The Zeiss Individual 2 uses Zeiss's Luminance Design technology, which adapts the lens design to the wearer's pupil size under different lighting conditions. The Zeiss Individual 2 also uses Zeiss's FrameFit+ technology, which adjusts the lens design to the wearer's frame parameters and facial anatomy. The Zeiss Individual 2 is available in three designs: Zeiss Individual 2 SV (single vision), Zeiss Individual 2 Near (near vision) and Zeiss Individual 2 Progressive (progressive vision).

Hoya: Hoyalux iD MyStyle V+

Hoyalux iD MyStyle V+ from Hoya, claims to be the first personalized progressive lens that adapts to the wearer's lifestyle and preferences. The lens design is based on an individualized 3D eye model that takes into account the wearer's eye shape, pupil size, and eye rotation. The lens also incorporates the wearer's personal wearing parameters, such as frame size, shape, and position, as well as the wearer's viewing habits, such as reading distance, head posture, and eye movement patterns. The result is a tailor-made progressive lens that provides a clear and comfortable vision for any activity and environment (Hoya Vision Care, 2021).

The benefits of AI-Designed Progressive Addition Lenses

The benefits of AI-designed progressive lenses are evident in terms of visual quality, comfort, and satisfaction. Several studies have shown that AI-designed progressive lenses can improve the visual acuity, contrast sensitivity, depth perception, and stereopsis of presbyopic patients compared to conventional progressive lenses. Furthermore, AI-designed progressive lenses can reduce the visual fatigue, eye strain, headache, and dizziness that are often associated with multifocal lens wear. Additionally, AI-designed progressive lenses can enhance the aesthetic appearance and self-confidence of the wearers by providing a more natural look and feel.

The drawbacks of AI-Designed Progressive Lenses

However, AI-designed progressive lenses are not without drawbacks. One of the main demerits of AI-designed progressive lenses is their high cost, which may not be affordable for all patients. Another potential disadvantage is the complexity of the fitting process, which requires more precise measurements and adjustments than conventional progressive lenses. Moreover, some patients may still experience some adaptation issues or dissatisfaction with their AI-designed progressive lenses due to individual differences or unrealistic expectations.

The Comparison

To compare different progressive lens designs versus AI-designed progressive lenses, it is important to consider several criteria, such as optical quality, visual fields, adaptation time, subjective comfort, patient satisfaction, and cost-effectiveness. Based on these criteria, AI-designed progressive lenses generally outperform conventional progressive lenses in most aspects. However, the choice of the best progressive lens design for each patient depends on their specific needs and preferences, as well as on the availability and accessibility of the products.

The Conclusion

In conclusion, AI-designed progressive lenses are a new paradigm in vision correction that offers a personalized and customized solution for presbyopic patients who need multifocal correction. By using advanced algorithms and data analysis, AI-designed progressive lenses can optimize the lens surface according to each wearer's factors and provide a wider and clearer field of vision at all distances. AI-designed progressive lenses are available in India and several other countries under different brand names and features. The benefits of AI-designed progressive lenses include improved visual quality, comfort, satisfaction, and appearance. The demerits of AI-designed progressive lenses include high cost, complex fitting processes, and possible adaptation issues or dissatisfaction.

References:

Alvarez, T L., Kim, E H., & Granger-Donetti, B. (2017, May 31). Adaptation to Progressive Additive Lenses: Potential Factors to Consider. https://scite.ai/reports/10.1038/s41598-017-02851-5

Boutron, I., Touizer, C., Pitrou, I., Roy, C., & Ravaud, P. (2008, September 19). The VEPRO trial: A cross-over randomised controlled trial comparing 2 progressive lenses for patients with presbyopia. https://scite.ai/reports/10.1186/1745-6215-9-54

Cagnie, B., Meulemeester, K D., Saeys, L., Danneels, L., Vandenbulcke, L., & Castelein, B. (2017, March 16). The impact of different lenses on visual and musculoskeletal complaints in VDU workers with work-related neck complaints: a randomized controlled trial. https://scite.ai/reports/10.1186/s12199-017-0611-1

Cai, H., Xu, J., Xiao, J., Zhang, Y., & Shi, G. (2017, June 1). Study on optical freeform surface manufacturing of progressive addition lens based on fast tool servo. https://scite.ai/reports/10.1088/1755-1315/69/1/012130

Carreño, E., Carreño, R., Carreño, M., López, V., & Potvin, R. (2020, February 1). <p>Refractive and Visual Outcomes After Bilateral Implantation of a Trifocal Intraocular Lens in a Large Population</p>. https://scite.ai/reports/10.2147/opth.s238841

Elmadina, A E M. (2022, July 21). Progressive addition lenses wearers' visual satisfaction among Saudi population. https://scite.ai/reports/10.4102/aveh.v81i1.733

Grzeszkowiak, J., & Wierzbowska, J. (2022, June 30). Choosing the right surgical treatment for hyperopia. https://scite.ai/reports/10.24292/01.ot.120622

Imburgia, A., Gaudenzi, F., Mularoni, K., Mussoni, G., & Mularoni, A. (2022, January 24). Comparison of clinical performance and subjective outcomes between two diffractive trifocal intraocular lenses (IOLs) and one monofocal IOL in bilateral cataract surgery. https://scite.ai/reports/10.31083/j.fbl2702041

Javidi, B., Carnicer, A., Arai, J., Fujii, T., Hua, H., Liao, H., Martínez-Corral, M., Pla, F., Stern, A., Waller, L., Wang, Q H., Wetzstein, G., Yamaguchi, M., & Yamamoto, H. (2020, October 12). Roadmap on 3D integral imaging: sensing, processing, and display. https://scite.ai/reports/10.1364/oe.402193

Palomino-Bautista, C., Cerviño, A., Cuiña-Sardiña, R., Carmona-González, D., Castillo-Gómez, A., & Sánchez-Jean, R. (2022, May 31). Depth of field and visual performance after implantation of a new hydrophobic trifocal intraocular lens. https://scite.ai/reports/10.1186/s12886-022-02462-3

Radhakrishnan, A., Dorronsoro, C., Sawides, L., & Marcos, S. (2014, March 24). Short-Term Neural Adaptation to Simultaneous Bifocal Images. https://scite.ai/reports/10.1371/journal.pone.0093089

Schilling, T., Ohlendorf, A., Varnas, S R., & Wahl, S. (2017, July 5). Peripheral Design of Progressive Addition Lenses and the Lag of Accommodation in Myopes. https://scite.ai/

reports/10.1167/iovs.17-21589

Song, K H., Choi, Y., & Lee, Y. (2019, July 23). A Study on the Deformation Behavior of a Microstructure Depending on Its Shape and the Cutting Section in the Precision Cutting of a Functional Part. https://scite.ai/reports/10.3390/app9142940

What ODs Should Know About the AI-Powered Varilux XR Lens. (n.d). https://eyesoneyecare.com/resources/ai-powered-varilux-xr-lens/

PROGRESSIVE LENSES STANDARD

Progressive lenses are a type of multifocal lenses that provide a smooth transition from distance to near vision without visible segments or lines. They are designed to correct presbyopia, a condition that affects most people over 40 and causes difficulty focusing on close objects. Progressive lenses have become increasingly popular due to their aesthetic appeal and functional benefits. However, not all progressive lenses are created equal. There are different types of progressive lens designs, each with its advantages and disadvantages. This book provides a brief overview of the main categories of progressive lens designs, such as conventional, free-form, personalised, digital, and AI-designed progressive lenses. It also explains the key factors that influence the performance and comfort of progressive lenses, such as the fitting parameters, the lens material, the coating, and the frame shape. The book aims to help optometrists, opticians, and eyewear consumers understand the basic principles and features of progressive lens designs and make informed choices when selecting or prescribing them.

www.ingramcontent.com/pod-product-compliance
Lightning Source LLC
LaVergne TN
LVHW051543170726
843492LV00006B/1919